Hematology

FOURTH EDITION

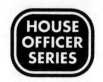

Hematology

FOURTH EDITION

Larry Waterbury, M.D.

Chief Hematology–Oncology Division
Johns Hopkins Bayview Medical Center
Associate Professor of Medicine and Oncology
The Johns Hopkins University School of Medicine
Baltimore, Maryland

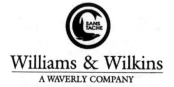

Williams & Wilkins
A WAVERLY COMPANY

BALTIMORE • PHILADELPHIA • LONDON • PARIS • BANGKOK
BUENOS AIRES • HONG KONG • MUNICH • SYDNEY • TOKYO • WROCLAW

Editor: Charles Mitchell
Managing Editor: Grace Miller
Production Coordinator: Anne Stewart Seitz
Designer: Dan Pfisterer
Cover Designer: Dan Pfisterer
Typesetter: Peirce Graphic Services, Inc.
Printer: Vicks, Inc.

Copyright © 1996 Williams & Wilkins
351 West Camden Street
Baltimore, Maryland 21201-2436 USA

Rose Tree Corporate Center
1400 North Providence Road
Building II, Suite 5025
Media, Pennsylvania 19063-2043 USA

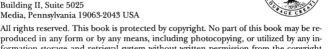

Accurate indications, adverse reactions and dosage schedules for drugs are provided in this book, but it is possible that they may change. The reader is urged to review the package information data of the manufacturers of the medications mentioned.

Printed in the United States of America

Library of Congress Cataloging-in-Publication Data

Waterbury, Larry, 1937–
Hematology / Larry Waterbury. — 4th ed.
   p.   cm. — (House officer series)
Rev. ed. of: Hematology for the house officer. 3rd ed. c1988.
Includes bibliographical references and index.
ISBN 0-683-08854-8
1. Blood—Diseases—Handbooks, manuals, etc.   2. Hematology—Handbooks, manuals, etc.   I. Waterbury, Larry, 1937– Hematology for the house officer. II. Title.
III. Series: The House officer series.
   [DNLM: 1. Hematologic Diseases—handbooks.   WH 39 W324h 1996]
RC636.W33   1996
616.1′5—dc20
DNLM/DLC
for Library of Congress   96-9114
                                                                                     CIP

To purchase additional copies of this book, call our customer service department at **(800) 638-0672** or fax orders to **(800) 447-8438.** For other book services, including chapter reprints and large quantity sales, ask for the Special Sales department.

Canadian customers should call **(800) 268-4178,** or fax **(905) 470-6780.** For all other calls originating outside of the United States, please call **(410) 528-4223** or fax us at **(410) 528-8550.**

Visit Williams & Wilkins on the Internet: http://www.wwilkins.com or contact our customer service department at **custserv@wwilkins.com.** Williams & Wilkins customer service representatives are available from 8:30 am to 6:00 pm, EST, Monday through Friday, for telephone access.

                                                                          96 97 98 99 00

1 2 3 4 5 6 7 8 9 10

To my wife Marcia,

my inspiration and the best

physician I know.

Preface

This 4th edition of Hematology (previously, Hematology for the House Officer) is designed to help students, house officers, internists and other primary care physicians logically evaluate patients with hematologic abnormalities. The focus is on differential diagnosis and diagnostic approaches to the more common hematologic problems encountered in a general medical practice. The esoteric, rare, and unusual are purposefully omitted to keep the physicians' focus limited to the most common and most likely diagnoses. Problems are grouped by clinical and laboratory presentation and designed to give the student/physician an organizational framework based on the actual way one encounters clinical problems of patients rather than by disease entity. For example, the chapters on anemia are organized based on variations in the routine database for all anemias (MCV, appropriateness of reticulocyte response, patient problem list, etc.). The chapters on coagulation abnormalities are organized by differential diagnosis based on the results of routine tests of hemostasis.

The book is designed to help physicians approach and, when appropriate, treat the most common hematologic problems faced in a general practice or admitted to a general hospital. When treatment is the appropriate responsibility of the generalist, with or without the guidance of the specialist, treatment sections are broadened and they are brief when treatment is best left to the specialist.

I have attempted to specifically address in a practical way the common questions posed to me by students, house officers and primary physicians using experience gained over many years of teaching and caring for patients with hematologic problems.

As in previous editions of this book I want to acknowledge and thank the many students and house officers I have known over the past 26 years here at Johns Hopkins Bayview Medical Center (formerly the Baltimore City Hospitals and the Francis Scott Key Medical Center), who through their questions and comments have helped in the formulation of this book.

As with previous editions, I have again been blessed with excellent clerical help from Mrs. Carole Messman.

LARRY WATERBURY, M.D.

About the Author

Dr. Waterbury is Chief, Division of Hematology–Oncology at Johns Hopkins Bayview Medical Center and Associate Professor of Medicine and Oncology at the Johns Hopkins University School of Medicine. He has authored many articles and chapters on Hematology and Oncology topics and is a contributor to a major textbook of ambulatory medicine. Principally a clinician with special interest in the longitudinal ambulatory care of general hematology and oncology patients, one of his major interests for many years has been the teaching of medical house officers and primary physicians.

Contents

Chapter 1

Anemia: Introduction and Approach to Diagnosis

ANEMIA: GENERAL CONSIDERATIONS

Normal hematocrit (HCT) and hemoglobin (Hgb) levels vary between laboratories and methods of determination. However, in general, anemia is present in adults when the HCT is reproducibly less than 42% in men or 37% in women or when the Hgb level is less than 14 g% in men or 12 g% in women. Most studies of normal values in the elderly reveal a slight decrease with aging (approximately 1–3% HCT points).

A number of in vivo and in vitro variables affect normal values and must be taken into consideration. Every house officer eventually encounters a puzzling HCT change in a newly admitted patient between the value obtained in the emergency room and the value obtained on the floor a few hours or a day later. Rather than bleeding or hemolysis, one or more of the following variables are usually to blame and are assessed by asking the following questions:

What is the state of the patient's hydration?

- HCT swings as high as 6–8% may occur with correction of dehydration or volume overload.

How was the blood specimen obtained?

- HCT/Hgb values are frequently higher from a finger, heel, or earlobe stick than from a venous sample unless excessive pressure is applied to facilitate blood flow, which lowers the hematocrit.

- Prolonged stasis from a tourniquet increases the hematocrit, as do muscular activity and cold.
- A drop of several HCT points may be seen between samples taken from a patient who is sitting and those taken after the patient has been lying down a few minutes as plasma volume increases when supine.

How was the HCT/Hgb determined?

If manual method, remember:

- Capillary tube HCTS are very reproducible (1–2% variability). Manual hemoglobin methods are less accurate.

Table 1.1
Hematocrit Variations throughout Life

	Hct %
Term newborn (cord blood)	44–62
Term newborn (capillary blood)	53–68
Infant (3 months)	30–38
Child (10 years)	37–44
Adult female	37–47
Pregnancy (30 weeks, gestation)	26–34
Adult male	42–54

Table 1.2
Variables Which Tend to Raise the Hematocrit

Dehydration
Finger stick (heel stick, earlobe) samples
Prolonged tourniquet stasis
Exposure to cold
Increased muscular activity
Upright position
Centrifugation techniques (especially with bizarre cell shapes)

Variables Which Tend to Decrease the Hematocrit

Volume overload
Supine position
Capillary tube leakage during centrifugation
Automated techniques

- Microhematocrits are frequently slightly higher than automated hematocrits (see below) because of plasma trapping (this is increased when red cells are misshapen, as in sickle cell disease and severe iron deficiency).
- Watch out for an occult leak from the poorly sealed capillary HCT tube.

If an automated method is used:

Most laboratories now use automated methods for the complete blood count (CBC). Routine data obtained usually include the HCT, Hgb, red cell count (RBC), mean corpuscular volume (MCV), mean corpuscular hemoglobin (MCH) and mean corpuscular hemoglobin concentration (MCHC). The following equations describe the relationships between these data:

$$MCV = HCT \div RBC \text{ (in cubic micrometers, or femtoliters, fl)}$$

$$MCH = Hgb \div RBC \text{ (in picograms, pg)}$$

$$MCHC = Hgb \div HCT \text{ (in grams/100 ml RBCs, g/dl RBCs)}$$

With automated systems the Hgb, RBC and MCV are directly measured and from these measured variables the HCT, MCH and MCHC are calculated. The major advantage of the automated system—other than the obvious advantages of speed, automated printout, etc.—is a high degree of reproducibility. The indices, especially the MCV, are precise values which can reliably be used in approaching the diagnostic workup of anemia. An additional dividend obtained from most automated machine CBCs is the red cell distribution width (**RDW**), a measure of the degree of variation in red cell size. Increased RDWs are a tip off to the

Table 1.3
Representative Normal Values

	Adult Male	Adult Female
Hgb (g/dl blood)	14–18	12–16
HCT (%)	42–54	37–47
MCV (fl)	82–98	82–98
MCH (pg)	27–32	27–32
MCHC (g/dl RBCs)	31.5–36	31.5–36

presence of qualitative red cell problems and identify the need for a competent review of a finger-stick smear.

The **MCV** is a measure of cell size and is more reproducible than one's ability to tell subtle changes in size from the examination of the peripheral smear. The **MCH** is a measure of the average amount of hemoglobin in each individual cell (essentially giving the same information as the MCV). The **MCHC** is a measure of the concentration of hemoglobin in each cell (a measure of chromicity).

HELP FROM THE PERIPHERAL SMEAR

The peripheral smear may give helpful and even definitive diagnostic information in the evaluation of anemia. Except at the extremes of cell size, the electronically measured MCV is superior to the peripheral smear in determining RBC size. However, RBC shape, chromicity, inclusions, etc. have definite diagnostic importance. Table 1.4 lists common conditions associated with various RBC morphologies.

ANEMIA: APPROACH TO WORKUP
Routine Database

The following is an appropriate routine database in the initial evaluation of anemia:

HCT
Hgb
MCV
MCHC
Reticulocyte count
Finger-stick peripheral smear

(The MCH gives essentially the same information as the MCV.)

Approach

Attempt to classify the anemia on the basis of (1) **cell size,** (2) **mechanism,** and (3) patient **problem list.** Answer the following three questions:

Table 1.4
Common Causes of Various RBC Abnormalities

Hypochromia, Microcytosis:	Iron deficiency
	Thalassemia
	Sideroblastic anemia
	Chronic inflammation
Macrocytosis:	Liver disease (central targeting)
	Megaloblastic anemia (macroovalocytes)
	Reticulocytosis
	Newborn
	Myelodysplastic syndromes (mimics megalo-blastic morphology)
	Myelophthysis
Marked Anisocytosis and Poikilocytosis: (variation in size and shape)	Marked iron deficiency
	Megaloblastic anemia (severe)
	Microangiopathic hemolysis
	Leukoerythroblastosis
	Hemoglobinopathies
Target Cells:	Liver disease
	C hemoglobin (AC, CC, SC)
	SS disease
	Postsplenectomy
	Thalassemia
	Artifact
Spiculated RBCs:	Hereditary acanthocytosis
	Liver disease (spur cells)
	Renal disease (burr cells)
	Postsplenectomy
	Hypothyroidism
	Microangiopathic hemolysis
Tear Drop Cells:	Leukoerythroblastosis
	Megaloblastic anemias
	Thalassemia
	Autoimmune hemolysis
Howell-Jolly Bodies:	Postsplenectomy
	Megaloblastic anemia
	Myelodysplastic syndromes
Pappenheimer Bodies:	Postsplenectomy
	Sideroblastic anemia
	Megaloblastic anemia
	Alcohol
	Marked hemolysis
	Thalassemia
Microspherocytes:	Hereditary spherocytosis
	Autoimmune hemolysis
	Hemoglobin C disorders (CC, SC)
	Severe burns
Ovalocytes:	Hereditary ovalocytosis
	Megaloblastic anemia
	Iron deficiency
	Thalassemia

1. **What is the MCV?**

The normal MCV varies depending on the method, but with automated methods is in the range of 82–98 fl. It is helpful to use a broad normal range of 80–100 fl to classify the anemia as **microcytic** (MCV < 80 fl), **normocytic** (MCV = 80–100 fl), or **macrocytic** (MCV > 100 fl).This is a most helpful step in the approach to etiology, since anemias with abnormal MCVs are caused only by a few conditions (Chapters 2 and 3).

2. **What is the basic mechanism of the anemia?**

There are three basic ways that anemia may develop:

- Decreased effective marrow **production**
- **Bleeding**
- **Hemolysis**

The following observations help to define the mechanism:

a. **Reticulocyte Index.** The reticulocyte count is used to assess the appropriateness of the bone marrow response to anemia. It must be corrected for the anemia to give a value known as the reticulocyte index (p. 36). Anemia with an appropriate bone marrow response (reticulocytosis) suggests bleeding or hemolysis. Be aware that a recently treated production-type anemia (e.g., iron deficiency) or the discontinuation of marrow suppression (e.g., withdrawal of alcohol) will also manifest appropriate reticulocytosis and mimic hemolysis or acute bleeding.

b. The **rate of HCT fall** may help in the assessment of the mechanism. Total marrow shutdown of RBC production in the absence of bleeding/hemolysis will result in an HCT fall of no greater than 3–4 HCT points per week (1/120 of the red cell mass per day, since the normal red cell survival is around 120 days). A more rapid fall, in the absence of marked plasma volume changes, usually means bleeding or hemolysis.

Remember: anemia with an appropriate reticulocyte response in the absence of bleeding suggests the presence of hemolysis.

3. What anemias are associated with the problems noted on the **problem list?**

For this purpose, race and sex should be considered as well. Women are frequently iron deficient; African American patients

Table 1.5
Anemias Associated with Various Clinical States

Female:	Iron deficiency
African-American:	G-6-PD deficiency, hemoglobinopathies, thalassemia
Mediterranean Origin:	G-6-PD deficiency, thalassemia
Far East Origin:	Hemoglobinopathies, thalassemia
Viral Infection:	Immune hemolysis, decreased production
Bacterial Infection:	Anemia of inflammation
	Microangiopathic hemolysis
	Oxidative hemolysis (G-6-PD deficiency)
	Other hemolytic mechanisms
Malignancy:	Anemia of chronic disease
	Microangiopathic hemolysis
	Immune hemolysis
	Decreased production
Alcoholic Liver Disease:	Bleeding
	Hypersplenism
	Folate deficiency
	Ethanol depression of production
	Sideroblastic anemia
	Iron deficiency
	Hemolysis
Hypothyroidism:	Decreased production
	Pernicious anemia
	Iron deficiency
Renal Failure:	Decreased production (low erythropoietin)
	Hemolysis
	Bleeding
	Marrow fibrosis (2^0 hyperparathyroidism)
Mechanical Aortic Valve:	Microangiopathic hemolysis
Malignant Hypertension:	Microangiopathic hemolysis
Rheumatoid Syndromes:	Anemia of chronic disease
	Iron deficiency
	Autoimmune hemolysis
Collagen Vascular Diseases:	Autoimmune hemolysis
	Anemia of chronic disease
Drugs:	Hemolysis
	Methyldopa (Aldomet): Immune hemolysis
	Quinine/quinidine: Immune hemolysis
	Penicillin: Immune hemolysis (rare)
	Sulfonamides; Immune, G-6-PD hemolysis
	Gold: Aplastic anemia
	Phenytoin (Dilantin): Megaloblastic anemia (folate), pure red cell aplasia
	Mitomycin: Microangiopathic hemolysis
	AZT: Decreased production
	Trimethoprim: megaloblastic anemia

may have hemoglobinopathies or hemolysis secondary to glucose-6-phosphate dehydrogenase (G-6-PD) deficiency. Table 1.5 lists some recognized causes for anemia in various clinical disease states.

SUMMARY

Classification on the basis of (1) **MCV,** (2) categorization of probable **mechanism,** and (3) consideration of possible cause raised by the **problem list** should then suggest further appropriate diagnostic evaluation.

Suggested Reading

Gulati GL, Hyun BH. The automated CBC, a current perspective. Hematology/Oncology Clinics of North America, August, 1994;8:593–603.

Williams WJ, Morris MW, Nelson DA. Examination of the blood. In: Beutler EB, Lichtman MA, Coller BS, Kipps TJ, eds. Williams Hematology. 5th ed. New York: McGraw-Hill, 1995:8–15.

Chapter 2

Anemia with a Low MCV

Commonly an MCV < 80 fl limits the anemia to one of two diagnoses: **iron deficiency** or some type of **thalassemia.** The anemia of chronic disease may occasionally be associated with an MCV in the 70s but usually is normocytic. Some hemoglobinopathies, most commonly hemoglobin E (Hgb E), are associated with a low MCV. It is seen almost exclusively in Southeast Asia, specifically Thailand, Cambodia, Malaysia and Indonesia. Sideroblastic anemias are characterized by heterogenous red cells, including a population of microcytic and hypochromic cells, but the MCV is rarely decreased and frequently increased (Chapter 5). Aluminum toxicity seen in some patients with chronic renal failure is an uncommon cause of mild microcytosis.

DIFFERENTIAL DIAGNOSIS

- Iron deficiency
- Thalassemia
- Anemia of chronic disease (Chapter 5)
- Some hemoglobinopathies (e.g., Hgb E)
- Sideroblastic anemia (congenital, MCV rarely low, Chapter 5)
- Aluminum toxicity

IRON DEFICIENCY ANEMIA

Dietary iron deficiency anemia may develop in infants and adolescents because growth needs outstrip dietary supply. In some countries inadequate diets cause dietary iron deficiency anemia in adults as well. However, in the United States, iron deficiency on the basis of diet alone in an adult is uncommon. In adults one should always assume that iron deficiency is secondary to blood loss. Iron deficiency in a man means gastrointestinal (GI) bleeding until proven otherwise. Many women are iron deficient because of menstrual bleeding or pregnancy. Patients with chronic **intravascular hemolysis** (such as microangiopathic hemolysis secondary to a mechanical aortic valve) may develop iron deficiency from iron loss in the urine. Patients with **pulmonary hemosiderosis** may develop iron deficiency from bleeding in the lung.

History

The following historical data suggest iron deficiency:

- Any menstruating woman, especially with past pregnancies.
- Pica: ice, starch, clay ingestion.
- Postgastrectomy for bleeding without adequate postoperative iron supplementation. Also decreased iron absorption secondary to achlorhydria.
- Any past history of GI bleeding.

Physical Findings

Sore tongue, cheilosis, brittle and ridged fingernails, spoon nails, and splenomegaly are all features of severe and long-standing iron deficiency anemia but are seen infrequently. Iron deficiency is associated rarely with an esophageal web and dysphagia (Plummer-Vinson syndrome, Patterson-Kelly syndrome).

The MCV (and MCH) are Usually Low

When blood loss occurs slowly but consistently over months, progressive anemia develops once the reticuloendothelial iron stores (approximately 1 g of iron in an adult) have been depleted. Initially red cell size and shape are unaffected, but as the anemia progresses cells become smaller and, later, misshapen. Generally the **MCV** and degree of poikilocytosis (variation in shape) correlate with the degree of anemia (Table 2.1). The **RDW** increases in severe iron deficiency anemia.

Table 2.1
Correlation of HCT, MCV and Shape Changes in Iron Deficiency Anemia

HCT (%)	MCV (fl)	Poikilocytosis
35	82	0
30	79	1+
25	74	2+
20	70	3+
15	65	4+

The MCV Can Be Normal

- Early, mild iron deficiency anemia.
- When blood loss occurs rapidly over days to weeks, the bone marrow can produce normocytic red cells while iron stores are adequate. Therefore, the MCV will often be normal despite a low hematocrit during early blood loss.
- Combined deficiencies of iron plus folate or B_{12}.
- Early iron deficiency in patients with macrocytosis of liver disease.

The MCHC Is Usually Normal

Hypochromia develops as the anemia increases. However, the MCHC (a measure of red cell chromicity) does not drop until the hematocrit is quite low (Table 2.2). RBCs on smear may appear hypochromic with a normal MCHC.

Other Diagnostic Aids In Iron Deficiency

- **Serum iron (SI).** Classically low, but also low in acute and chronic inflammation and malignancy. The SI may fall within a matter of hours at the onset of acute infection. Other variables affect the SI including time of day (peak between 7 and 10 AM, nadir around 9 PM), Menstruation (decreases), following acute MI (decreases), oral iron R_x (increases in a few hours), Parenteral iron R_x (increased for weeks).
- **Total iron-binding capacity (TIBC).** A measure of transferrin in terms of the amount of iron it can bind, the TIBC is classically elevated but is actually normal in many patients with iron deficiency. It is low in chronic inflammation and malignancy.

- **Transferrin saturation (TS).** Usually less than 16% in iron deficiency, but may be just as low in acute or chronic inflammation. Useful in the diagnosis of iron deficiency mainly in the setting of an elevated TIBC. If greater than 25%, iron deficiency is unlikely.

- **Reticulocyte index.** Inappropriately low for the degree of anemia (p. 36).

- **Serum ferritin.** A low level invariably indicates iron deficiency. May be spuriously normal in several clinical settings (Table 2.3).

- Bone **marrow iron stain.** Absent iron stores in iron deficiency. The major exception occurs in patients treated recently with parenteral iron. A percentage of the iron accumulates in the marrow but is unavailable for hemoglobin production. Also, after transfusion one may see bone marrow iron in patients who are still iron deficient. Sometimes with the anemia of chronic disease, small amounts of marrow iron may be seen in patients with iron deficiency anemia.

- **Peripheral smear.** In early iron deficiency the smear is usually normal. It is difficult to pick up early subtle changes in cell size in early iron deficiency (microcytosis precedes poikilocytosis) and the MCV is more helpful than the smear at this stage. In severe iron deficiency anemia there is marked poikilocytosis and hypochromia without stippling. Elliptical ("cigar-shaped") cells are common. The few young cells seen on the smear frequently appear as polychromatophilic target cells.

- **RDW.** Usually elevated in severe iron deficiency. May help distinguish iron deficiency from heterozygous thalassemia (RDW usually normal, may be elevated).

- **Free erythrocyte protoporphyrin (FEP).** Elevated after iron deficiency is present for several weeks and returns to normal only after weeks to months of iron therapy. Mainly used for screening for iron deficiency in infants.

- Miscellaneous. Either **thrombocytosis** (common) or mild thrombocytopenia as well as leukopenia may occasionally be seen in severe iron deficiency anemia.

- **Drop in MCV.** One of the most helpful observations in the diagnosis of iron deficiency is a low MCV which previously

Table 2.2
Representative Data Bases at Various Stages in the Slow Development of Severe Iron Deficiency Anemia

HCT	42	42	35	27	19
MCV (82–98 fl)	92	88	81	75	68
MCHC (32–36 g/dl)	33	33	33	33	29
SI (65–175 µg%)	70	60	35	20	20
RDW (11.5–14.5%)	13	13	14	15	17
TIBC (250–375 µg%)	300	300	300	400	450
Serum ferritin (10–200 µg/L)	60	20	5	3	1
Peripheral smear	Normal	Normal	Normal	1+ poikilocytosis 1+ hypochromia	4+ poikilocytosis 4+ hypochromia
Bone marrow iron stores	Present	Absent	Absent	Absent	Absent

(months or years before) was normal. In thalassemia a low MCV is life-long. In the absence of chronic inflammation a drop in MCV almost always means iron deficiency.

Common Appropriate Database

Most iron deficiency anemias may be diagnosed on the basis of **history,** the **MCV, peripheral smear,** and the **serum ferritin** concentration.

The Serum Ferritin

The serum ferritin is a useful measure of reticuloendothelial iron stores and essentially provides the same clinical information as a bone marrow iron stain. Between the ranges of 20 μg/L and 200 μg/L, one μg/L serum ferritin represents 10 mgm storage iron. The serum ferritin increases with age.

The ferritin remains low for 2–3 weeks when patients are started on usual doses of oral iron (e.g., 60 mg elemental iron bid), then increases and can no longer be used to monitor iron deficiency in treated patients. Following parenteral iron therapy the serum ferritin will rise within 24 hours of the first injection and persist for several months.

The major problem with the serum ferritin as a diagnostic test for iron deficiency is that it is spuriously elevated in a number of clinical settings. Table 2.3 lists conditions associated with serum ferritin levels which frequently are inappropriately high for the amount of reticuloendothelial iron present. Under these

Table 2.3
Inappropriately Normal or Elevated Serum Ferritin Levels

Acute liver disease
Cirrhosis
Hodgkin's disease
Acute leukemias
Solid tumors (occasional)
Fever
Inflammation
Chronic renal failure (dialysis)
Parenteral iron
Oral iron (2–3 wks into Rx)

conditions, patients with iron deficiency anemia may have normal or even elevated serum ferritin levels.

In patients with the anemia of chronic disease, serum ferritin can be used sometimes to distinguish those who are iron deficient as well. However, the normal range may have to be adjusted upward as inflammation may elevate the serum ferritin level in iron-deficient patients. The same applies to hemodialysis patients. A number of studies of dialysis patients and patients with inflammation have demonstrated that a serum ferritin less than 50–60 µg/L is highly suggestive of iron deficiency.

Treatment Tips

Standard medical therapy consists of one oral iron tablet (there are 60 mg of elemental iron in one 300 mg $FeSO_4$ tablet) tid on an empty stomach (1 hour before meals). Long-term treatment may be needed (6 months in a man, 1 year in a menstruating woman) to replenish iron stores. Avoid time-release capsules and enteric coated preparations as absorption is variable. The addition of ascorbic acid to aid absorption is not effective enough to be worth the cost. Although iron absorption is decreased in patients with achlorhydria or patients who are postgastrectomy, treatment with oral iron is still usually successful. In patients on histamine H_2 receptor (H_2) blockers absorption is decreased primarily from iron complexing with the medication, not achlorhydria. Patients should take iron and **H_2 blockers** separately. **Omeprazole** may also inhibit iron absorption.

Patient compliance is the major problem with oral iron therapy. Approximately 15% of patients have GI side effects from oral iron (cramping, constipation, diarrhea). The following compromises may help compliance:

1. Bid treatment rather than tid. The middle of the day dose is difficult for patients to take.
2. Once a day for a year is better than bid or tid for 6 weeks.
3. If GI side effects occur, try the following:
   a. Administer the iron with meals (decreases absorption 50%), but not with **antacids** or with **tea** (markedly decreases absorption).

    b. If symptoms persist, decrease the size of each dose to less than 40 mg elemental iron (ferrous gluconate tabs [38 mg], ferrous sulfate syrup [45 mg/tsp], or ferrous sulfate pediatric drops [25 mg/ml]).

4. Parenteral iron (**iron dextran,** 50 mg/ml) is rarely necessary if the above compromises are tried. Parenteral iron is indicated in patients with small and large bowel inflammation, rapid transit GI problems, malabsorption, and proven noncompliance. There is no solid evidence that parenteral iron can accomplish a more rapid hematocrit response than oral iron. In fact, after the first week of therapy, evidence shows that the response lags behind that achieved by oral therapy.

Side effects from parenteral iron include:

    a. Intramuscular (usual dose: 2 ml deep IM/day).
- Pain at the injection site
- Staining of the skin
- Fever
- Exacerbation of arthritis
- Anaphylaxis (very rare but should only be given in a setting where treatment for anaphylaxis is available. Test dose required before the first injection.)

    b. Intravenous (usual dose (1–2 ml IV daily).
- Fever
- Exacerbation of arthritis
- Anaphylaxis (see above)
- Local phlebitis if diluted with D5W
- Hypotension if administered faster than 50 mg (1 ml)/minute.

Treatment Response

The maximal reticulocyte response is seen 7–10 days following initiation of oral iron therapy. Reticulocyte counts on either side of the peak reticulocyte response may not be very high, especially if the anemia is not severe. The hematocrit will begin to rise 7–10 days following initiation of treatment at a rate inversely proportional to the degree of anemia. It takes 1–3 months to normalize the hematocrit in uncomplicated iron deficiency anemia.

THALASSEMIA

The thalassemias are inherited defects in globin chain production resulting in microcytic anemia and are seen primarily (in the United States) in African American, Mediterranean (Greek or Italian), and Asian patients. Most patients are heterozygotes and have mild, usually clinically asymptomatic anemias, but sometimes marked red cell microcytosis. Diagnosis is important to distinguish thalassemia from iron deficiency (patients are frequently worked up repetitively for iron deficiency and treated with iron) and for genetic counseling.

Typical Routine Database Results
for Heterozygous Thalassemia

Hematocrit	37
MCV	69
MCH	21
RDW	14
MCHC	33
Reticulocytes	3%

Smear: microcytosis; moderate anisocytosis and poikilocytosis; occasional target cells, ovalocytes and occasionally coarsely stippled red cells.

This database should stimulate the following question:

Why Is the MCV So Low for Such a Mild Anemia?

This should suggest a diagnosis of heterozygous thalassemia. Typically, the **MCV** is in the 70s (occasionally 60s) but the hematocrit is normal or only slightly decreased. In iron deficiency an MCV this low is usually seen only with moderate to severe anemia (Table 2.2, p. 13). The occasional heavily **stippled red cell** on peripheral smear is also helpful in differentiating thalassemia from iron deficiency. Such cells are more common in Greek or Italian patients than in African American patients with thalassemia. The **RDW** reported with CBCs done on automatic counters is a measure of variation in red cell size. It has reportedly been a useful measure to distinguish heterozygous thalassemia from iron deficiency. However, there is considerable overlap. Whereas almost all patients with severe iron deficiency anemia have an elevated RDW, most heterozygous thalassemia patients do not; 20 to 40% of patients with heterozygous thalassemia have an elevated RDW as well. An elevated **red cell count** is also characteristic of heterozygous thalassemia.

The polycythemic patient with iron deficiency may have a database which mimics heterozygous thalassemia. This is common in polycythemia vera patients.

Differential Diagnosis

1. Thalassemia
2. Polycythemia with iron deficiency

Additional Database Information

Three major hemoglobins are present in mature red cells of normal adults. Each hemoglobin molecule consists of four heme groups and four globin chains. There are two different types of globin chains in each hemoglobin molecule. The following table shows that these hemoglobins share one type of common globin chain (α chains), but differ in second globin chain type (β, δ, γ):

Hemoglobin	%	Globin chain type
A	97	$\alpha 2\beta 2$
A_2	2	$\alpha 2\delta 2$
F	1	$\alpha 2\mu 2$

Hemoglobin electrophoresis. There is decreased production of β globin chains in heterozygous β-thalassemia resulting in a decreased production of hemoglobin A, and a compensatory increase in δ globin chain production resulting in an increase of Hgb A_2 (4–6%).

Assay of Hgb F. In heterozygous β-thalassemia there may also be a compensatory increase in production of γ globin chains, resulting in an increase of Hgb F (2–8%, present in about 50% of patients).

Miscellaneous. Other test results may help to distinguish thalassemia from iron deficiency: normal or elevated **serum ferritin;** the presence of iron on a bone **marrow iron stain;** normal or elevated **SI;** the **RBC count;** and the **RDW.**

What If Thalassemia Is Suspected but Hgb A_2 Is Not Increased?

Possible Explanations

1. Concomitant **β-thalassemia and iron deficiency** (the reason for the reduction of A_2 Hgb is not clear).

2. **β-δ-thalassemia.** This syndrome commonly results in a slightly more severe anemia, a normal or low hemoglobin A_2, and an increased hemoglobin F.

3. **α-thalassemia.** Heterozygous β-thalassemia is the most common form of thalassemia seen in American white populations usually of Mediterranean background. Heterozygous α-thalassemia is more common in African Americans affecting approximately 25% of the population. α Chains are present in all three normal adult hemoglobins. Therefore, decreased α globin chain production does not alter the ratio of the three adult hemoglobins. Diagnostic proof of α-thalassemia requires specialized research techniques such as restriction endonuclease mapping. There are four genes (found on paired chromosomes 16) which code for α chain production as compared to two genes (found on paired chromosomes 11) which code for β chain synthesis. Various α chain syndromes are described in Table 2.4 below.

Table 2.4
α Thalassemia Syndromes

Genotype	Terminology	Clinical Features
αα/α-	Heterozygous α-thalassemia 2 present in 25% of American Blacks. Only a portion are clinically identifiable (low MCV, MCH)	Normal or Thal trait
αα/—	Heterozygous α-thalassemia 1; very rare in African Americans	Thal trait
α-/α-	Homozygous α-thalassemia 2; 2–3% of African Americans	Thal trait
α-/—	Hemoglobin H disease. Very rare in African Americans because of the rarity of α-thalassemia 1	Thal intermedia
—/—	Homozygous α-thalassemia 1	Hydrops fetalis

Clinical Management

- **Patient education.** Explain that the clinical features mimic iron deficiency and that patients should be on guard to protect themselves from iron deficiency workups. Emphasize the benign nature of the illness in heterozygotes. Explain that the anemia, being mild, does not usually cause symptoms (an Hct of 35% does not explain fatigue). Caution against taking oral iron.

- **Genetic counseling.** A couple, both heterozygous for β-thalassemia, have a 25% chance of having a child with homozygous thalassemia major ("Cooley's anemia"). The gene defects for β-thalassemia and those for Hgb S and Hgb C are alleles. Hgb S-β-thalassemia is a clinically significant disease. The presence of heterozygous or homozygous α-thalassemia 1 in patients with SS or SC disease seems to ameliorate the clinical severity of those syndromes. It is now possible to make a prenatal diagnosis of some of the above syndromes by amniocentesis.

- **Thalassemia major.** These patients require specialized treatment and should be followed by physicians experienced in their care.

Suggested Reading

Cook JD, Skibne BS. Iron deficiency: definition and diagnosis. J Intern Med 1989;226:349.

Fairbanks VF, Beutler EB. Iron deficiency. In: Beutler EB, Lichtman MA, Coller BS, Kipps TJ, eds. Williams Hematology, 5th ed. New York: McGraw-Hill, 1995:490–511.

Johnson CS, Tegos C, Beutler E. Alpha-thalassemia. Prevalence and hematologic findings in American Blacks. Arch Intern Med 1982; 142:1280.

Schwartz E, Benz EJ,Forget BG. Thalassemia syndromes. In: Hoffman R, Benz EJ, Shattil SJ, Furie B, Cohen HJ, Silberstein LE, eds. Hematology: Basic Principles and Practice. 2nd ed. New York: Churchill Livingstone, 1995:586–610.

Chapter 3

Anemias with a High MCV

An MCV greater than 100 fl requires an explanation. The differential diagnosis of the common etiologies is short. Some causes, such as marked reticulocytosis and macrocytosis seen in the newborn, are obvious from the routine database. Further diagnostic studies may be necessary to distinguish megaloblastic anemia from a myelodysplastic syndrome or from severe liver disease, as well as to define the specific etiology of a megaloblastic anemia once that diagnosis is made. The following is a list of common causes of an MCV greater than 100 fl. A number of these causes are not associated with anemia.

DIFFERENTIAL DIAGNOSIS OF AN MCV GREATER THAN 100 FL

1. Spurious
2. Reticulocytosis (marked)
3. Liver disease
4. Alcoholism
5. No associated disease
6. Myelodysplastic syndromes
7. Drugs
8. Megaloblastic anemias
9. Pregnancy (MCV rises, rarely >100 fl)
10. Hypothyroidism (MCV rises, rarely >100 fl)
11. Rare miscellaneous causes

1. A number of technical factors may contribute to a **spurious** elevation of the MCV measured by electronic counters.

These include low temperature and inadequate removal of the bleach solution used to clean the system. Marked hyperglycemia or chronic hypernatremia will result in cell swelling when cells are placed in the more hypotonic counting solution. High titer "cold" red cell autoantibodies may on occasion, by agglutination, cause spuriously high MCVs. Sometimes a markedly elevated white count will raise the MCV as larger white cells are confused for red cells by the electronic counter.

2. Young red cells are large and will elevate the average MCV. Reticulocyte counts usually must be very high to increase the MCV over 100 fl. It is uncommon to see an MCV greater than 115 fl from **reticulocytosis** alone.

3. Hepatocellular and obstructive **liver disease** is frequently associated with an elevated MCV (usually less than 115 fl). In liver disease the red cell membrane accumulates lipid. The cells appear large, round, and targeted on smear, without the marked variation in size and shape characteristic of megaloblastic anemia. This morphologic abnormality is not an explanation for anemia, although patients with liver disease frequently have anemia from other mechanisms.

4. Even without evidence of liver disease or a megaloblastic anemia, the alcoholic patient frequently has a mildly elevated MCV (100–110 fl). There is a correlation between the degree of elevation of the MCV and the amount of **alcohol** consumption. The MCV level decreases slowly (2–4 months) on discontinuation of alcohol intake.

5. Occasionally one sees a mild elevation of the MCV (100–105 fl) in a patient **without any known cause** and it may be normal.

6. Many patients with **myelodysplastic syndromes** (idiopathic sideroblastic anemia, refractory anemia with an excess of blasts, etc., p. 24) have a macrocytic anemia with an elevated MCV. The MCV is usually less than 115 fl, but occasionally can be as high as levels seen in severe megaloblastic anemias (e.g., in the 5q- syndrome).

7. A number of **drugs** cause mild to severe megaloblastic bone marrow changes with associated peripheral macrocytosis. Alcohol and diphenylhydantoin interfere with folate use and/ or absorption. Methotrexate and trimethoprim bind to dihydro-

folate reductase, interfering with folate metabolism. Other chemotherapeutic agents, such as cytosine arabinoside and hydroxyurea, interfere with DNA metabolism, resulting in a hematologic defect that mimics folic acid deficiency. Chronic use of cyclophosphamide, 6-mercaptopurine, azathioprine, 5-fluorouracil and other chemotherapeutic agents results in a mild elevation of the MCV.

8. **Megaloblastic anemia** (p. 26).

9. The MCV frequently rises during **pregnancy,** even in patients without folate deficiency. Rarely does the MCV exceed 100 fl.

10. An elevated MCV in **hypothyroidism** should trigger a search for pernicious anemia. In the absence of B_{12} deficiency the MCV rises in some hypothyroid patients but usually does not exceed 100 fl. The MCV drops slowly with thyroid replacement.

11. **Miscellaneous** causes include some patients with aplastic anemia and pure red cell aplasia present with a mild macrocytosis. Bone marrow malignancies such as myeloma, lymphoma, metastatic cancer, and other causes of marrow crowding, may demonstrate a peripheral macrocytosis.

HINTS REGARDING ETIOLOGY FROM THE INITIAL ROUTINE DATABASE

Common Historical and Physical Findings

- Sore tongue, smooth tongue (megaloblastic anemia)
- Peripheral neuropathy, dorsal column signs, "megaloblastic madness," corticospinal track signs (rarely), hypothyroidism or hyperthyroidism, post-total gastrectomy, ileal disease or resection (B_{12} deficiency).
- Alcoholic, marked inanition, malabsorption, phenytoin (folic acid deficiency or inhibition).
- Stigmata of liver disease.

Routine Laboratory Help

- An **MCV greater than 115 fl** is unusual except in megaloblastic anemia.
- Marked variations in red cell size (**anisocytosis**) and shape (**poikilocytosis**) with **ovalocytes** on smear are classically seen in

severe megaloblastic anemia but may also be seen in the myelodysplastic syndromes.

- **Leukopenia** and **thrombocytopenia** are common in megaloblastic anemia and myelodysplasia but might also be seen in liver disease for different reasons (hypersplenism, alcohol).
- The **reticulocyte count** is inappropriately low in megaloblastic anemias and myelodysplasia.
- Neutrophil **hypersegmentation** is common, although not invariable, in megaloblastic anemias. It is not seen in myelodysplasia. This helps to distinguish the two syndromes which may present similar peripheral blood findings.
- Bizarre **platelet morphology** and **qualitative white cell changes** favor a diagnosis of myelodysplasia.
- The macrocytes in liver disease are round and frequently **targeted,** not oval as in megaloblastic anemia.

ADDITIONAL DATABASE INFORMATION

If the etiology of the elevated MCV is not obvious after the above considerations, subsequent diagnostic workup is indicated. That workup is initially directed at evaluation for the presence of a megaloblastic anemia and consists of:

1. Serum B_{12} assay
2. RBC folate assay
3. Bone marrow

This data should distinguish a megaloblastic anemia from the syndrome of myelodysplasia, which may mimic a megaloblastic process.

Table 3.1
FAB Classification of the Myelodysplastic Syndromes

Refractory anemia (RA)
Refractory anemia with ringed sideroblasts (RARS)
Refractory anemia with excess of blasts (RAEB)
Chronic myelomonocytic leukemia (CMML)
Refractory anemia with excess of blasts in transition (RAEB-T)

THE MYELODYSPLASTIC SYNDROMES

These syndromes are a result of an acquired bone marrow stem cell disorder and are seen primarily in older patients. Frequently there are qualitative and quantitative abnormalities of all cell lines, and the picture may mimic closely a megaloblastic anemia. The MCV does not reach the levels seen in severe megaloblastic anemias and usually is less than 110 fl. The MCV may be normal. On peripheral smear review red cells typically exhibit marked anisocytosis and poikilocytosis with macro-ovalocytes and stippling. Nucleated red cells may be seen. Leukopenia and thrombocytopenia may be present. Platelets may appear large and degranulated and there may be qualitative white cell changes and an increase in young mononuclear cells. Hypersegmentation of the polys is not seen. The bone marrow usually is hypercellular with qualitative changes in all cell lines. Erythrocyte precursors appear megaloblastic ("megaloblastoid"). White cell precursors usually reveal a left shift and are abnormal with clusters of young mononuclear forms. The iron stain frequently reveals ringed sideroblasts. The serum B_{12} and serum folate levels are frequently elevated and there is no response to folic acid or B_{12} treatment. With time (months to sometimes several years) such patients usually slowly develop a picture of acute leukemia.

Historically these syndromes were known as preleukemia, smoldering leukemia, erythroleukemia and Di Guglielmo's syndrome. In recent years they have been more clearly defined with more functional semantics by the FAB (French-American-British) classification listed in Table 3.1. Chromosome studies are also helpful in classification and definition of prognosis in these syndromes.

Treatment

Refractory anemia (RA) and refractory anemia with ringed sideroblasts (RARS) have the best prognoses of the myelodysplastic syndromes. If the anemia is mild, observation alone is appropriate, but progression to transfusion dependence is the rule. Pyridoxine and folic acid are tried in RARS (helpful in some cases of congenital sideroblastic anemia, and some cases of drug-induced sideroblastic states) but almost always are ineffective. Androgen

Table 3.2
Causes of Vitamin B$_{12}$ Deficiency

Dietary (strict vegan's diet—rare in the US, usual vegetarian diet won't cause)
Gastric intrinsic factor abnormality (pernicious anemia, total gastrectomy)
Terminal ileum disease (ileal resection or bypass, Crohn's disease, sprue)
Competition for intestinal B$_{12}$ (fish tapeworm infestation, bacterial overgrowth, as in blind loop syndrome)
Pancreatic insufficiency (abnormal Schilling test, but only rarely causes clinical disease
Drugs interfering with absorption (colchicine, alcohol, but they don't cause clinical disease)
Congenital (transcobalamin II deficiency, Imerslund syndrome)

treatment is often tried but only occasionally helpful. Erythropoietin plus granulocyte, or granulocyte-macrophage colony stimulating factor (G-CSF, GM-CSF), may eliminate transfusion dependence for a variable period of time in up to 40% of patients, but is expensive; the combination is more effective than erythropoietin alone. Chelation with desferrioxamine is indicated as iron overload is common and may cause death.

MEGALOBLASTIC ANEMIA

Tables 3.2 and 3.3 list the various causes of vitamin B$_{12}$ and folic acid deficiency.

Table 3.3
Causes of Folic Acid Deficiency or Inhibition

Decreased **intake** (alcoholism, starvation)
Increased **loss** (psoriasis, dialysis)
Increased **requirement** (pregnancy, infancy, chronic hemolysis)
Decreased **absorption** (sprue, Crohn's disease, small bowel lymphoma or amyloidosis)
Drugs:
  Inhibition of dihydrofolate reductase (methotrexate, trimethoprim)
  Purine analogs (azathioprine)
  Pyrimidine analogs (Zidovudine)
  RNA reductase inhibitors (hydroxyurea)
  Miscellaneous [phenytoin (Dilantin), N$_2$]

History and Physical Examination

Remember that **pernicious anemia** (PA) is by far the most common etiology of B_{12} deficiency. It is more common in northern Europeans, especially Scandinavians. It is also common in African Americans, especially women, where it is frequently severe on presentation and seen at a younger age than the norm (7th decade). The body's store of B_{12} will last for years, and, therefore, dietary B_{12} deficiency is extremely rare. Patients may complain of sore mouth, indigestion, constipation or diarrhea. When anemia is severe they may have a pale lemon-yellow color to their skin, a combination of anemia plus a mild increase in bilirubin. **Neuropsychologic problems** (Table 3.4) such as peripheral neuropathy, dorsal column signs, and changes in affect are common. Anemia develops so slowly that patients may be acclimated to very low hematocrits. Other causes of B_{12} deficiency are listed in Table 3.2. After total gastrectomy or total ileectomy, all patients will, after several years (average 5–6 years), develop B_{12} deficiency and megaloblastic anemia. These patients should receive prophylactic B_{12} treatment. After partial **gastrectomy** a patient only occasionally develops B_{12} deficiency (5%). Twenty-five to 50% of gastrectomy patients may have a low B_{12} level and an abnormal Schilling test, but clinical disease is uncommon. In **Zollinger-Ellison syndrome,** the marked hyperacidity may interfere with transfer of B_{12} from protein binders to intrinsic factor leading to clinically significant B_{12} deficiency.

In contrast to B_{12} deficiency, the body's stores of folic acid will last only a few weeks, therefore, **folic acid deficiency** is usually dietary in etiology. Folic acid deficiency is seen most commonly in the alcoholic or the patient with extremely poor food intake, for any cause, of several weeks' duration. The condition is also seen in

Table 3.4
Neurologic Features of B_{12} Deficiency

Peripheral neuropathy	Common
Dorsal column signs	Relatively common
Corticospinal tract signs	Rare
"Megaloblastic madness"	Common

pregnant women not taking folic acid supplements, and rarely in the patient with hemolysis. The symptoms are those of B_{12} deficiency but without the neurologic manifestations. Folic acid deficiency as a cause of neuropsychiatric problems is controversial. The alcoholic may have a neuropathy from alcohol.

Laboratory

Peripheral Blood and Bone Marrow. Peripheral blood and bone marrow morphology is the same in B_{12} and folic acid deficiency with moderate-to-severe anemia. In severe deficiency the **MCV** may be greater than 115 fl. The **RDW** is increased; the reticulocyte count is inappropriately low. If the anemia is severe, red cells demonstrate marked **anisocytosis** and **poikilocytosis,** with **macro-ovalocytes.** There may also be small misshapen cells. **Howell-Jolly bodies, Pappenheimer bodies,** and nucleated RBCs may be seen. The neutrophils are frequently hypersegmented (occasional six or more lobed cell) and decreased in number. Note: A left shift in granulocytes, as with infection, or severe neutropenia may mask hypersegmentation. **Hypersegmentation** usually persists for 10 days to 2 weeks after treatment. Platelets are frequently decreased. Bone marrow is typically hypercellular with megaloblastic changes of erythroid and granulocytic precursors. The iron stain of the marrow frequently reveals abnormal sideroblasts, and occasional ringed sideroblasts may be seen. Megaloblastic changes occur in other cells in the body including GI tract epithelial cells. Abnormal PAP smears occur and may suggest malignancy.

Serum Folate and B_{12} Levels. In B_{12} deficiency (**PA**), the serum B_{12} level is low and the serum folate level is usually normal or elevated. The RBC folate level may be artificially low. Following one injection of B_{12} the serum B_{12} level may be elevated for weeks, eliminating it as a diagnostic tool for B_{12} deficiency. The serum B_{12} level may be elevated in chronic myeloproliferative syndromes because of the presence of increased levels of binding proteins. The B_{12} level is false in a number of clinical settings (see Table 3.5).

In megaloblastic anemia due to **folic acid deficiency** the serum folate is typically low. However, the serum folate is so sensitive to recent dietary intake that it is of little help in the diagnostic workup

Table 3.5
Serum B$_{12}$ Assay

May be spuriously low when tissue stores are normal
- Some patients with folate deficiency (30–50%
- Sometimes in pregnancy (25%
- Vegetarians
- High daily doses of Vitamin C
- Congenital transcobalamin I (TCI) deficiency

May be spuriously normal when tissue stores are deficient
- Acute megaloblastic anemia due to N_2O
- Congenital transcobalamin II (TCII) deficiency
- Myeloproliferative syndromes (elevated TCI

RBC Folate Assay
1. Reflects chronic folate deficiency
2. Falsely low in some patients with B$_{12}$ deficiency
3. Falsely high in reticulocytes

Serum Folate Assay
1. A measure of recent dietary intake of folate
2. Usually normal or elevated in B$_{12}$ deficiency

of megaloblastic anemia. The red cell folate is a better indicator of chronic folate deficiency, remaining low for the life of the cell. The serum B$_{12}$, although usually normal, may be low in up to 30% of patients with folate-deficient megaloblastic anemia. The low B$_{12}$ level is not because of a deficiency of B$_{12}$ and normalizes within a few days after beginning treatment with folic acid.

Table 3.6
Differentiating Between Folate and B$_{12}$ Megaloblastosis

Etiology by History	RBC Folate	Serum B$_{12}$	Interpretation	Further Testing
Suggests folate	↓	Nl or ↑	Folate deficiency	None
Suggests folate	↓	Sl ↓	Folate deficiency	Recheck B$_{12}$ after folate Rx for 1 week
Suggests B$_{12}$	Nl or ↑	↓	B$_{12}$ deficiency	None
Suggests B$_{12}$	↓ (serum folate usually ↑)	↓	B$_{12}$ deficiency	May confirm with Schilling test

All other combinations Schilling test.

Table 3.7
Causes of a Falsely Positive Schilling Test

1. Incomplete urine collection
2. Renal failure
3. Some patients with megaloblastic anemia before treatment
4. Gastric antibodies to intrinsic factor
5. Defective intrinsic factor
6. Drugs (alcohol, colchicine, neomycin, potassium, cholestiramine)
7. Pancreatic insufficiency
8. Partial gastrectomy

Falsely normal Schilling tests may be seen after other isotope studies, e.g., gallium, tech-nechium.

Schilling Test

The Schilling test is of use primarily in cases in which there is confusion about the etiology of a megaloblastic anemia. The test requires a cooperative patient who can and will collect 24-hour urine samples. The Schilling test may be abnormal initially in megaloblastic anemias (including folate deficiency) because of intestinal mucosal cell dysfunction secondary to the megaloblastic process. The Schilling test is more reliable after the megaloblastic anemia has been treated for 1–2 weeks. Table 3.7 lists problems encountered with interpretation of the Schilling test.

Serum Methylmalonic Acid and Homocysteine

Increasingly recognized are patients with subtle clinical manifestations consistent with B_{12} deficiency who have non-diagnostic serum B_{12} assays and Schilling tests. Many patients are elderly and without hematologic features of megaloblastosis, but have neuropsychiatric features of B_{12} deficiency. Such patients may be identified by elevated serum levels of methylmalonic acid and homocysteine, sensitive indicators of tissue B_{12} deficiency. Such patients may malabsorb food-bound B_{12}, but absorb free B_{12} (as administered in the Schilling test) adequately. Many of these patients have borderline low B_{12} levels. Serum methylmalonic acid and homocysteine assays are complicated, expensive, and not cost effective in most clinical situations. Thus it may be reasonable to institute a therapeutic trial of B_{12} in patients with unexplained neurologic findings consistent with B_{12} deficiency, subtle or no suggestive hematologic features, and borderline serum B_{12} levels.

Other Laboratory Features

Megaloblastic anemias are **hemolytic** in the sense that there is marked intramarrow destruction of abnormally formed red cells (**ineffective erythropoiesis**). There is frequently **indirect hyperbilirubinemia,** elevated serum lactate dehydrogenase (**LDH**), and an elevated serum iron as in other hemolytic states. There is gastric achlorhydria in pernicious anemia. The **reticulocyte index** is inappropriately low. In PA **antibodies** to gastric mucosal cells and intrinsic factor (IF) are commonly found in the serum as well as antithyroid and antiadrenal antibodies. **Serum anti-IF antibodies** are present in 65–70% of patients with PA and because of its high degree of specificity, is a helpful test in the diagnosis.

Treatment

B_{12} deficiency. One hundred micrograms of intramuscular B_{12} administered monthly is adequate therapy for most patients. Occasionally patients may require 200 μgms monthly. Many physicians will treat patients daily while they are in the hospital, especially if neurologic manifestations are prominent. However, there are few data to indicate that this is helpful. Monthly injections for life are indicated for patients with PA, after total gastrectomy, or with terminal ileum disease. Serum potassium may fall during the first few days of B_{12} therapy for severe megaloblastic anemia; some experts recommend monitoring and potassium replacement.

Folic Acid Deficiency. One milligram P.O. daily is adequate treatment for most patients. Alcoholics may require 5 mg daily. Pregnant women, hemodialysis patients, and patients with severe hemolytic states should receive 1 mg per day of prophylactic folic acid. Replacement may be particularly important in pregnancy where folate deficiency has been linked to neural tube defects in newborns. However, the defects occur within the first few weeks of pregnancy before a woman may even know she is pregnant. Folic acid administration will not interfere with the efficacy of methotrexate treatment in psoriasis and may help to prevent megaloblastosis (folinic acid is the treatment for methotrexate toxicity). Most data suggest little difference in efficacy if folate is given for phenytoin-induced megaloblastosis; some data suggests folate, especially in high doses, can cause a decrease in seizure threshold, and folic acid should probably not be given prophylactically.

With appropriate treatment of B_{12} and folic acid deficiency, there is a rapid reticulocytosis that reaches its peak at about 7 days. The height of the reticulocyte response depends on the severity of the anemia. When the hematocrit is very low, the reticulocyte response may be 30 or 40% in the absence of other processes which blunt bone marrow response (inflammatory illness, etc.). The leukopenia and thrombocytopenia usually respond within a few days. In PA, "megaloblastic madness" usually corrects rapidly; dorsal column disease and peripheral neuropathies usually improve, but more slowly. Corticospinal tract signs are usually permanent.

Transfusion. Some patients with a megaloblastic process may develop a very severe anemia. This is especially common in pernicious anemia. Resist the temptation to transfuse the elderly PA patient because the hematocrit is 10 to 15%. Such patients have developed the anemia very slowly and frequently are well compensated (have adjusted to changes including an expanded total blood volume). Transfusion, even of packed cells, may precipitate pulmonary edema. If comfortable at bedrest, it is best, if possible, to treat with the appropriate vitamin (and bedrest, or both if the etiology is not clear), and avoid the hazard of transfusion. If transfusion is necessary (see below) consider exchange transfusion to prevent increasing the blood volume, or concomitant treatment with diuretics.

Major Indications for Transfusion

1. Angina
2. Ischemic changes on electrocardiogram
3. High output heart failure

Suggested Reading

Beck WS: Diagnosis of megaloblastic anemia. Annual Review of Medicine 1991;42:311–322.

Goasguen JE, Bennett JM. Classification and morphologic features of the myelodysplastic syndromes. Seminars in Oncology 1992;19:4.

Greenberg PL. Treatment of MDS with hemopoietic growth factors. Sem Oncol 1992;19:106–114.

Savage D, Lindenbaum J, Stabler SP, Allen RH. Sensitivity of serum methylmalonic acid and total homocysteine determinations for diagnosing cobalamin and folate deficiencies. Am J Med 1994;96:239.

Stabler SP, Allen RH, Savage DG, Lindenbaum J. Clinical spectrum and diagnosis of cobalamin deficiency. Blood 1990;76:871–881.

Chapter 4

Hemolysis and Bleeding: Anemia with a Normal or Slightly Elevated MCV and an Appropriate Reticulocyte Index

Anemia resulting from hemolysis or bleeding is characterized by the presence of a reticulocytosis indicating an appropriate bone marrow response. The MCV is usually normal, although a mild elevation is not uncommon when the **reticulocyte count** is significantly elevated (p. 22). A reticulocyte count is used to assess the appropriateness of the bone marrow response to the anemia and should be part of the routine database. **Anemia with an appropriate reticulocyte response in the absence of overt bleeding suggests hemolysis.**

Recall that:

1. The normal reticulocyte count in a patient with a normal HCT is 1%. Approximately 1% (20 ml of RBCs per day in an adult) of circulating RBCs are removed daily and replaced by marrow reticulocytes.
2. The marrow can triple its production of RBCs almost immediately in response to acute blood loss or hemolysis.
3. If hemolysis is chronic over months or years, the marrow pro-

duction may reach a level of production greater than 10 times normal.

RETICULOCYTE INDEX

For the reticulocyte count to be used as an indicator of marrow responsiveness, it must be corrected for anemia. This corrected reticulocyte count is known as the reticulocyte index.

$$\text{reticulocyte index} = \text{reticulocyte \%} \times \frac{\text{patient HCT}}{\text{normal HCT}}$$

In anemia, with the same amount of bone marrow production, the percentage of reticulocytes increases because the reticulocytes are diluted in fewer red cells. This gives a false impression of increased bone marrow responsiveness. When the bone marrow response to anemia is appropriate, the reticulocyte index is at least 3%.

$$\text{HCT 10\%} \qquad \text{reticulocyte count 5\%}$$
$$\text{reticulocyte index} = 5\% \times \frac{10}{50} = 1\%$$

In this example, which uses an arbitrary normal Hct of 50% for ease of calculation, an inappropriately low reticulocyte index indicates that bone marrow production is at least a contributing factor in the etiology of anemia. The elevated reticulocyte count of 5% is misleading. For this degree of anemia an appropriate reticulocyte count would be at least 15%:

$$\text{reticulocyte index} = 15\% \times \frac{10}{50} = 3\%$$

THE "SHIFT" PHENOMENON

Young, very large reticulocytes or "shift cells," which ordinarily remain in the bone marrow 2 or 3 days before release, are shifted out of the marrow early into the peripheral blood when the anemia is severe and develops rapidly. This phenomenon explains the very high reticulocyte counts in acute and marked anemias. High reticulocyte counts, especially when many shift cells are present, may result in an elevated MCV.

Think of Hemolysis When

1. Anemia is accompanied by an appropriate reticulocyte index in the absence of evidence of bleeding. But recognize the following **pitfalls:**
   a. Patients with production anemias (as in iron deficiency, folate deficiency, alcoholism, and infection) will sometimes experience severe reticulocytosis in response to treatment (iron, folate, ethanol withdrawal, antibiotics), resulting in a laboratory database that may mimic hemolysis.
   b. There may be silent internal blood loss (e.g., retroperitoneal bleeding in a patient on anticoagulation, or bleeding at the site of a hip fracture) which may mimic hemolysis. Bleeding is much more common than hemolysis. Always suspect occult bleeding. Recognize the total amount of blood loss through phlebotomy that may occur during prolonged hospitalization.
2. Hemolysis is also suggested by a hematocrit that falls rapidly over a few days in the absence of bleeding. If red cell survival is normal, complete shutdown of marrow production results in a hematocrit drop at a normal rate of only 3–5 points per week. A faster rate of fall suggests bleeding or hemolysis.

Approach to Hemolysis

Before any attempt to define the specific etiology, it is reasonable first to try to prove hemolysis as the mechanism for the anemia. Additional appropriate diagnostic tests will vary depending on whether one suspects an intravascular or extravascular mechanism.

Intravascular Hemolysis (Table 4.1)

When RBC destruction is rapid and occurs primarily within the vascular space, diagnosis is relatively easy. One sees the following:

1. **Hemoglobinemia:** Although one may measure the plasma hemoglobin level directly, visual inspection alone is useful. Plasma serum becomes visibly red or brown at a low level of

Table 4.1
Clinical States Associated with Intravascular Hemolysis

1. Acute hemolytic transfusion reactions
2. Severe and extensive burns
3. Physical trauma (e.g., March hemoglobinuria)
4. Severe microangiopathic hemolysis (e.g., mechanical aortic valve pros thesis)
5. Acute G-6 -PD hemolysis
6. Paroxysmal nocuturnal hemoglobinuria
7. Clostridial sepsis

Hgb (around 30 mg%), a level that occurs from the lysis of only a few milliliters of red cells. Simple screening tests for hemoglobin (e.g., Hemoccult) are too sensitive to be helpful in this determination as there is normally a low level of free plasma hemoglobin from the trauma of drawing and centrifuging blood.

2. **Hemoglobinuria** occurs once haptoglobin (see below) is saturated. Hgb-haptoglobin complex is too large to pass the glomerulus and is cleared by the reticuloendothelial system and may be suspected by visual inspection of the urine (red or brown). Occult blood in the urine in the absence of any microscopic hematuria suggests hemoglobinuria but does not distinguish it from myoglobinuria. Because myoglobin is a small molecule, it freely passes through the glomerulus resulting in red or brown urine without plasma coloration. The larger hemoglobin molecule accumulates in the plasma before passing into the urine, resulting in red or brown coloration of both.

3. Saturation of **haptoglobin** is a binding protein for hemoglobin produced in the liver, occurs rapidly with an appreciable hemoglobinemia. Measurement of free haptoglobin is, therefore, a useful test in hemolysis. However, results may not be available for several days.

4. **Hemosiderinuria** is iron seen within renal tubular cells on an iron stain of the urinary sediment, is seen several days after the hemolytic event. Free hemoglobin containing iron passes the glomerulus and is absorbed by renal tubular

cells, which slough, appear in the urine several days later and stain positively for iron.

Thus an appropriate further database when hemolysis is suspected in the above clinical settings would include:

1. Observation of the serum/plasma.
2. Observation of the urine.
3. Measurement of free plasma hemoglobin.
4. Heme pigment test of the urine if there are no red cells in the urine sediment.
5. Measurement of free serum haptoglobin.
6. Iron stain of urine sediment for hemosiderin several days after a presumed hemolytic event.

Do not forget the help that may be obtained from the peripheral smear (p. 40).

Extravascular Hemolysis (Table 4.2)

Most hemolytic events do not take place intravascularly. When destruction occurs primarily within phagocytic cells of the reticuloendothelial system (RES), diagnosis is more difficult. There is no hemoglobinemia, hemoglobinuria, or hemosiderinuria. Haptoglobin is only partially saturated; there is a slight leak of free hemoglobin into the circulation, even when hemolysis primarily occurs extravascularly. There may be an indirect hyperbilirubinemia (insensitive) and an increase in the urine urobilinogen (unreliable). Red cells are rich in lactate dehydrogenase (LDH), which is frequently elevated in the serum. However, the test is nonspecific.

Table 4.2
Common Clinical States Associated with Extravascular Hemolysis

1. Autoimmune hemolysis
2. Delayed hemolytic transfusion reactions
3. Hemoglobinopathies
4. Hereditary spherocytosis
5. Hypersplenism
5. Hemolysis with liver disease

The RBC survival is shortened, but this test is tedious and takes days to complete. In short, the physician must often be satisfied with only presumptive evidence of extravascular hemolysis. When extravascular hemolysis is suspected, it is appropriate to move on to diagnostic tests of specific hemolytic states based on possible etiologies from the problem list and baseline data base without absolute proof of hemolysis. Most clinical hemolytic states are associated with extravascular hemolysis.

Help from the Peripheral Smear

- Frequently the smear reveals only **evidence of bone marrow response** (polychromatophilia, "shift cells," fine, diffuse stippling).
- Occasionally individual red cell morphology suggests an etiology, but frequently the morphology is normal. **There is no such thing as a "hemolytic smear."** When present, the following cell types are helpful:

1. **Spherocytes**
   In small numbers, these are seen in many different etiologies. In large numbers, they suggest the following:
   a. Hereditary spherocytosis.
   b. Autoimmune hemolysis.
   c. Hgb C hemoglobinopathies (CC, SC, C-thalassemia).
2. **Elliptocytes/ovalocytes**
   Hereditary elliptocytosis.
3. **Fragmentation (schistocytes)**
   Sharply pointed poikilocytes (helmet cells, spiculated cells, triangle cells) seen in microangiopathic hemolytic states (p. 49).
4. **Spiculated cells (acanthocytes, echinocytes)**
   Sometimes seen in patients with severe liver disease and hemolysis (usually seen only in patients with end-stage, terminal liver disease). Also, one of the types of schistocytes seen in microangiopathic hemolysis.
5. **"Bite" cells (keratocytes)**
   Cells sometimes seen in patients with oxidative hemolysis (e.g., G-6-PD deficiency with hemolysis). In such cells all of the hemoglobin appears to be pushed to one side of the cell.
6. **Poikilocytosis of the hemoglobinopathies** (Ch. 6).

HEMOLYSIS WITH A POSITIVE COOMBS' TEST

Once the physician suspects hemolysis from the above considerations, further diagnostic exploration should be guided by the
routine data base and the problem list. Because of the common
occurrence of immune hemolysis and the important therapeutic
implications of this diagnosis, a Coombs' test is frequently obtained at this point if the etiology is not apparent.

Positive Coombs' Test: Serologic Questions

The serologic questions raised by finding a positive direct
Coombs' test are the following:

1. **What exactly is on the surface of the red cell causing the positive test?**

   A screening direct Coombs' test usually employs **nonspecific
   Coombs' antiserum** harvested from animals immunized with
   whole human serum, which will cause red cell agglutination if
   any one of a number of serum constituents is present on the cell.
   Specific Coombs' antisera allow the blood bank technician to distinguish among the following possibilities:

   a. **Transferrin:** Present on the surface of reticulocytes; there-
      fore, marked reticulocytosis may cause a weak positive di-
      rect Coombs' test with the use of broad-spectrum Coombs'
      antiserum. The direct Coombs' test using specific anti-IgG
      or anti-C3 will be negative.

   b. **Nonspecific protein binding:** Sometimes seen in patients
      receiving high doses of cephalosporins (negative Coombs'
      with specific antisera).

   c. **Complement:** Present in many cases of antibody-induced
      hemolysis. Complement may be present without an iden-
      tifiable antibody. Its presence implies the presence of an-
      tibody no longer on the red cell or present in too low a
      concentration to identify.

   d. **Antibody:** For the most part these are IgG antibodies, as
      Coombs' antisera do not contain anti-IgM or anti-IgA in
      significant concentration.

2. **If antibody is present or presumed (complement alone), is it
   an alloantibody or an autoantibody?** (Table 4.3)

Table 4.3
Alloantibody versus Autoantibody

	Alloantibody	Autoantibody
Direct Coombs'	Frequently negative. May be positive if sensitized foreign red cells are still circulating	Positive
Indirect Coombs' Antibody Screen (Panel)	Positive Specificity is seen	Positive or negative Panagglutination, no specificity seen

Alloantibodies

- Induced by exposure to foreign red cells (transfusion or through pregnancy).
- Directed against specific minor red cell antigens.
- Present in the serum and identified by an **antibody screen** (indirect Coombs' test).
- Present on red cells (positive direct Coombs' test) only when transfused or fetal red cells are circulating, having been sensitized but not yet destroyed.

The blood bank can identify the specificity of such antibodies by the pattern of reactivity seen using the patient's serum and a panel of red cells of known and variable individual antigenicity. Alloantibodies react only with the cells containing the guilty antigen as opposed to the pan-reactivity of autoantibodies. Occasionally the blood bank reports a positive antibody screen due to a naturally-occurring antibody. Such antibodies are not induced by prior exposure to foreign red cells but may be quite hemolytic if incompatible blood is transfused (e.g., anti-A, anti-B, and antibodies of the Lewis and P blood groups).

Clinical Significance. It is crucial to identify the presence and specificity of alloantibodies to assure the safety of future transfusions. The difficulty of finding compatible blood relates to the prevalence of the specific offending antigen or antigens. The physician must communicate closely with the blood bank to understand the problems the technician faces in finding compatible blood.

Autoantibodies

A positive direct Coombs' test due to an antibody in a nonpregnant and not recently transfused patient is almost always due to an inappropriately produced autoantibody (immunologic defect, cross-reacting antibody secondary to drugs, infection, etc.). When eluted off the red cells, or if present also in the serum, the antibody reacts as a **pan-agglutinin,** reacting with all the cells in a routine red cell panel, making cross matching impossible.

3. Once it is determined that the positive direct Coombs' test is due to an autoantibody, the next **serologic question** is whether the antibody is a "warm antibody" or a "cold antibody."

   a. **Warm Antibody**
   • Usually IgG. Cannot be identified by direct agglutination (requires Coombs' test for identification).
   • Some IgG antibodies fix complement. Specific Coombs' antisera testing may reveal IgG alone, IgG plus C3 or, sometimes C3 alone.

   b. **Cold Antibodies or "cold agglutinins"**
   • Usually **IgM** and can be identified by direct agglutination in the cold. (Does not require Coombs' test for identification).
   • Positive **"bedside cold agglutination test."** Clumping may be seen by tilting a tube of the patient's anticoagulated blood in front of a light after placing it in a cup of ice water for 5 minutes.
   • Cold hemolysins (**Donath-Landsteiner antibody**) are rare in adults (seen in tertiary syphilis) but may be the cause of virus-induced hemolysis in children.
   • Positive Coombs' test due to **C3 alone** (positive "nongamma" Coombs' test). IgM fixes C3 on the cell in the cold or at room temperature. IgM falls off on warming, but the C3 remains attached to the cell.
   • Elevated **cold agglutinin titer.** A low titer of naturally oc-

curring cold agglutinins is normal. An elevated titer, read microscopically, is usually greater than 1:32. Sera should be separated from the red cells immediately after drawing the blood while it is still warm in order not to lose antibody from adherence to the red cells as the blood cools to room temperature.

* The antibody usually is directed against a ubiquitous red cell antigen known as "I." Occasionally cold agglutinins, for example, those seen commonly in infectious mononucleosis, have a specificity for red cell antigen "i," which is present on newborn red cells.

Positive Coombs' Test: Clinical Questions

The clinical diagnostic and therapeutic considerations depend on the answers to the serologic questions discussed above.

AUTOIMMUNE HEMOLYSIS AS A RESULT OF A "WARM ANTIBODY"
Differential Diagnosis

A. Idiopathic
B. Secondary
  Acute:
      Infection (particularly viral)
      Drugs
          Methyldopa (Aldomet)
          Penicillin
          Quinine/quinidine type
          Many other drugs rarely
  Chronic:
      Collagen vascular disease [systemic lupus erythematosus (SLE)]
      Lymphoproliferative disorders
      Miscellaneous (thyroid disease, malignancy, etc.)

Idiopathic Autoimmune Hemolysis (IAIH)

Some patients with IAIH subsequently develop diseases known to be associated with autoimmune hemolysis, such as SLE or lymphoma.

Peak age of onset is the 7th decade. Patients usually present with symptoms of anemia. The physical examination may reveal a slightly enlarged spleen in 50% of cases. Mild jaundice may be seen. The peripheral smear typically reveals polychromatophilia with "shift cells" and spherocytes. Usually the reticulocyte count is elevated; however, reticulocytopenia may be present in as many as 1/3 of patients. There is often a neutrophilia, but the WBC and platelet counts may be normal or slightly decreased. Rarely, severe autoimmune thrombocytopenia (Evan's syndrome) may be present as well.

Secondary Autoimmune Hemolysis

Acute, self-limited cases may be associated with various viral illnesses or secondary to a number of drugs. Several different mechanisms have been described in hemolysis secondary to drugs.

1. Methyldopa (Aldomet)

Seen in patients on large doses of methyldopa for several months. Usually there is only a positive Coombs' test without hemolysis. There is IgG alone on the surface of the red cell, and the serologic characteristics are exactly those seen in idiopathic (warm antibody) autoimmune hemolysis. The hematocrit returns to normal after the drug is discontinued, although the direct Coombs' test may remain positive for months. In the absence of hemolysis, methyldopa may be continued in patients with a positive Coombs' test alone.

2. Quinine/quinidine type

Rare, but when seen usually presents with a fulminant hemolysis which may follow soon after initiation of treatment. Antibody induced by the drug combines with the drug, and the immune complex deposits on the red cell. This is the mechanism for hemolysis with a large number of other drugs which even more rarely may produce hemolysis.

3. Penicillin

Again, rare and more often seen in patients on massive doses of penicillin. The drug adheres to the surface of the red cell, occasionally inducing the formation of a hemolytic antibody. Note that this is not the common, clinically unimportant, antipenicillin antibody present in most patients receiving the drug, and not the antibody responsible for penicillin reactions.

Chronic cases of **secondary** Coombs'positive hemolysis are seen in patients with(SLE) (where the hemolysis may precede diagnosis by months or years) and lymphoproliferative disorders [chronic lymphocytic leukemia (CLL), lymphosarcoma, or Waldenström's macroglobulinemia]. Rarely Coombs' positive hemolysis may be associated with other malignancies, hyperthyroidism, various bacterial infections, and immunodeficiency states.

AUTOHEMOLYSIS DUE TO COLD AGGLUTININS
Differential Diagnosis

1. Primary Cold Agglutinin Disease
2. Secondary
   a. Mycoplasma infections
   b. Viral infections
   c. Lymphoproliferative disease

The **primary** idiopathic form of the condition is rare. It is seen in elderly men with a monoclonal IgM serum protein electrophoretic spike. Symptoms may include ischemia of the ears, nose and fingers, in addition to anemia. Titers may be massively elevated.

Most commonly, cold agglutinin hemolysis is seen **secondary** to mycoplasmas or viral infections, SLE or lymphoproliferative diseases. Fifty percent of patients with mycoplasmas pneumonia will have an elevated cold agglutinin titer, but only a fraction of these have clinically significant hemolysis. Cold agglutinins (low titer with a specificity for the "i" antigen) are common in infectious mononucleosis, but significant hemolysis is rare.

COOMBS' NEGATIVE AUTOIMMUNE HEMOLYSIS

Up to 10% of patients with autoimmune hemolysis will have a negative direct Coombs' test. This is usually due to the insensitivity of the Coombs' test in identifying small numbers of antibodies on the red cell surface. Special techniques available in referral immunohematology laboratories can sometimes identify red cell antibodies. Patients with classic features of autoimmune hemolysis but a negative Coombs' test, after ruling out other possible causes of hemolysis, should be treated like Coombs'-positive hemolysis.

TREATMENT
Acute Autoimmune Hemolysis

Acute Coombs'-positive hemolysis related to mycoplasma or viral infections or to drugs usually requires only the discontinuation of the drug or time to recover from the infection.

Chronic Idiopathic Autoimmune Hemolysis (Warm Antibody)

Chronic Coombs'-positive hemolysis due to a warm antibody frequently responds to steroids. Prednisone in doses of 40–60 mg per day in divided doses (q.i.d.) is commonly employed (responses sometimes require higher doses of steroids). Response may take 1–3 weeks to occur. The prednisone is then tapered slowly over several weeks. Most patients may be tapered off the steroid or to a small daily dose (2.5–7.5 mg prednisone per day). When hemolysis is severe and unresponsive to steroids, or when the daily steroid dose is too high for safe long-term use, splenectomy should be considered. Danazol (anecdotal reports) may be useful in allowing a decrease in steroid dose and the avoidance of splenectomy. In addition, there are isolated case reports of responses to intravenous gamma globulin. Immunosuppressive agents such as azathioprine and cyclophosphamide are usually reserved for the patient refractory to steroids and splenectomy. There are isolated reports of the effectiveness of other treatments in refractory patients (e.g. 2-chloro deoxyadenosine). In many patients the disease is characterized by remissions and exacerbations over years.

Secondary Autoimmune Hemolysis (Warm Antibody)

Secondary autoimmune hemolysis due to a warm antibody (SLE, CLL, lymphoma) may be more refractory to treatment (steroids and splenectomy) and responds best to successful control of the underlying disease process.

Cold Agglutinin Hemolysis

Steroids and splenectomy are much less successful in cold agglutinin hemolysis, although they are usually attempted. Protection from the cold may be helpful in chronic idiopathic cold agglutinin disease.

Transfusion Therapy

Transfusions may be necessary in these patients, although problematic, as compatible blood may be impossible to find. One should avoid transfusion if possible, but, if necessary, transfusion with ABO- and Rh-compatible blood may be attempted with close observation of the patient. Although the survival of the transfused cells is not normal, severe, immediate intravascular hemolytic transfusion reactions are uncommon, and there may be temporary improvement in the hematocrit. Small daily transfusions may be safer and more successful than a single, large transfusion. In patients with cold agglutinins it is reasonable to use blood that has been warmed to body temperature and washed packed red cells to remove complement.

The major danger relates to the difficulty in identifying a dangerous alloantibody in the setting of a warm autoantibody. The blood bank should attempt to hunt for hidden alloantibodies, using special techniques (e.g., warm autoabsorption or a differential absorption technique). In addition, some warm autoantibodies have Rh specificity which is important to identify because transfused cells lacking the specific Rh antigen will survive longer.

Some patients present with a fulminant picture and may die from overwhelming hemolysis within hours. These patients need immediate transfusion. Such patients are frequently reticulocytopenic and they may have intravascular hemolysis with hemoglobinemia and hemoglobulinuria. Be wary of an altered consciousness, an accompanying acidosis, liver enzyme abnormalities, and red urine. Such patients need urgent transfusion in the ICU.

HEMOLYSIS WITH FRAGMENTED RED CELLS ON PERIPHERAL SMEAR

Microangiopathic Hemolytic Anemia (MAHA)

Differential Diagnosis

Mechanical aortic valve

Arteritis (malignant hypertension, polyarteritis, Scleroderma, etc.)

Disseminated intravascular coagulation (DIC)

Thrombotic thrombocytopenic purpura (TTP)

Hemolytic uremic syndrome (HUS)

Malignancy (mucin producing adenocarcinomas, especially cancer of the stomach)

Giant hemangiomas

Renal & hepatic transplant rejection

Eclampsia (preeclampsia, HELLP syndrome)

Chemotherapy (mitomycin, bleomycin)

Bone marrow transplantation (preceded by total body irradiation)

Cyclosporin A

Database

- The **peripheral smear** poikilocytosis is usually quite characteristic and may be differentiated from other conditions with marked poikilocytosis. The abnormal cells are sharply pointed and are called **schistocytes.** Common cell shapes include **helmet cells, triangle cells,** and **spiculated cells.**
- If **hemolysis** is severe it is usually **intravascular,** resulting in:
  Hemoglobinemia
  Hemoglobinuria
  Haptoglobin saturation
  Hemosiderinuria
  Iron deficiency if chronic (as with aortic valve prosthesis).
- If accompanied by significant thrombocytopenia, think of DIC, hemolytic uremic syndrome, TTP or severe eclampsia. Thrombocytopenia is destructive, so there should be ample bone marrow megakaryocytes and large platelet forms on a finger stick smear (p. 88).

HEMOLYSIS WITH AN ENLARGED SPLEEN

Although congestive splenomegaly is the most common cause, one may see cytopenias in patients with large spleens from any cause. All large spleens do not cause cytopenias, and the degree of cytopenia does not correlate with spleen size. Usually thrombocytopenia and leukopenia are more prominent than anemia. Red cell morphology is usually normal except for polychromatophilia and occasional spherocytes. Splenomegaly is sometimes seen in patients with hemolysis from other mechanisms (e.g., autoimmune hemolysis, hereditary spherocytosis, etc.). One almost never has to consider splenectomy for hypersplenic cytopenias. Some patients with **Felty's syndrome** complicated by recurrent infections from leukopenia are benefitted by splenectomy, as are patients with chronic leukemia or lymphomas.

HEMOLYSIS WITH LIVER DISEASE

Severe acute and chronic hepatocellular damage may be accompanied by hemolysis of unknown etiology. Occasionally one sees spiculated red cells (**"spur cells"**) on peripheral smear, a feature usually associated with severe hepatocellular disease and a very poor prognosis. Remember that patients with liver disease frequently have other mechanisms for anemia and reticulocytosis:

- Ethanol withdrawal may allow reticulocytosis in the alcoholic.
- A reasonable diet or folate replacement may result in a brisk reticulocytosis in the patient with alcoholic hepatitis and folate deficiency.
- Bleeding.
- Hypersplenism.

HEMOLYSIS WITH MICROSPHEROCYTES ON SMEAR
Differential Diagnosis

Hereditary spherocytosis (HS)
Coombs' positive hemolysis (p. 41)
Hemoglobin C disorders (Ch. 6)
Severe burns

Database

Spherocytes may be difficult to identify on peripheral smears and require some experience to differentiate from a common peripheral smear artifact. However, their presence in large numbers suggests one of the above diagnoses.

Hereditary Spherocytosis

This is a molecularly heterogenous, usually autosomal-dominant condition associated classically with microspherocytes, polychromatophilia, and a palpable spleen. Mild jaundice is common. Severity varies, and some cases are not recognized until later in life. The condition is caused by one of a number of inherited red cell membrane protein defects. In vitro autohemolysis in the absence of added glucose is accentuated, as is the osmotic fragility of the cells. **Splenectomy** often normalizes the hematocrit. **Hereditary elliptocytosis** is a similar group of disorders associated with peripheral elliptocytes. It is less frequently associated with significant hemolysis and represents more of a morphologic curiosity than a clinical problem.

ACUTE HEMOLYSIS IN PATIENTS WHO ARE AFRICAN AMERICAN OR OF MEDITERRANEAN OR ORIENTAL ETHNIC BACKGROUND

In African American, Mediterranean, and oriental populations, the presence of hemolysis raises the possibility of **G-6-PD deficiency, thalassemia** (p. 17), or a **hemoglobinopathy** (Ch. 6). Clearly G-6-PD deficiency occurs in patients other than African American, oriental, Greek or Italian in descent, and such patients may hemolyze for reasons other than for G-6-PD deficiency. However, it is worth focusing on the above association, as most patients with G-6-PD hemolysis in this country are African American, Mediterranean, or oriental.

Remember:

- 10% of African American males in the United States are affected (hemizygotes, sex-linked inheritance).
- 20% of African American females are heterozygotes (1% are homozygotes).
- In the African American patient, G-6-PD deficiency causes only an acute self-limited hemolytic anemia, whereas in the Mediterranean

Table 4.4
Common Drugs/Agents Implicated in G-6-PD Hemolysis

Sulfonamides
Sulfones
Primaquine phosphate
Nitrofurantoin
Phenazopyridine (Pyridium)
Fava beans

type, or one of the myriad of other G-6-PD mutations, hemolysis is more severe and one may see in these patients chronic ongoing compensated or partially compensated hemolysis, as well as hemolytic disease of the newborn.

- Hemolysis is precipitated usually by **infections** (bacterial, viral) or certain **drugs** (Table 4.4)
- Hemolysis is classically intravascular with transitory hemoglobinemia, hemoglobinuria and delayed hemosiderinuria.

Diagnosis

- One sometimes sees a characteristic cell on smear (**"bite cell,"** **"blister cell"**) at the height of the hemolysis (p. 40).
- **Screening tests** for the enzyme deficiency are not always positive:

  1. Around 30% of heterozygote females with African American G-6-PD deficiency have a normal G-6-PD screening test (**spot test**).
  2. Following hemolysis, when the affected cells have been destroyed, the heterozygote, especially with the African-type of enzyme deficiency, usually gives a normal screen and may not be diagnosable until G-6-PD-deficient cells (older cells) accumulate again in significant numbers in several weeks.
  3. In the African type, even the hemizygote male may have a normal screen following hemolysis. Although all of his cells are deficient, young cells have significant enzyme levels that drop only as cells age. A male with the Mediterranean type of deficiency is usually easily diagnosed even after hemolysis.

Typical Case

A young, previously healthy black woman presents with infectious hepatitis:

- HCT—19%
- Reticulocytes—18%
- Peripheral smear—polychromatophilia, "shift cells," and "bite cells"
- Urine hemoglobin is present in the absence of hematuria
- Haptoglobin is saturated
- Several days later the urine sediment stains positively for iron (positive urine hemosiderin test)
- G-6-PD screen normal
- G-6-PD screen 2 months later—positive for G-6-PD deficiency

Treatment

There is no specific treatment for the African type of G-6-PD deficiency other than avoidance of those drugs known to initiate oxidative hemolysis. Recovery from hemolysis is usually rapid. Rare cases of acute renal failure have been reported. Occasionally transfusion may be necessary. African-type G-6-PD deficiency patients are protected from repeat hemolysis until cells age and drop their enzyme levels, again becoming susceptible to an oxidative stress. In the Mediterranean type, and some of the more severe mutant enzyme types, hemolysis may be severe and chronic. Splenectomy may be required.

Suggested Reading

Engelfriet CP, Overbeeke MAM, von dem Borne AEG. Autoimmune hemolytic anemia. Seminars in Hematology 1992;29:3.

Rosse WF. Autoimmune hemolytic anemia. Hosp Pract 1985;20:105.

Schrier S. Extrinsic nonimmune hemolytic anemias. In: Hoffman R, Benz EJ, Shattil SJ, Furie B, Cohen HJ, Silberstein LE, eds. Hematology: Principles and Practice, 2nd ed. New York: Churchill Livingstone, 1995:729–736.

Schwartz RS, Silberstein LE, Berkman EM. Autoimmune hemolytic anemias. In: Hoffman R, Benz EJ, Shattil SJ, Furie B, Cohen HJ, Silberstein LE, eds. Hematology: Principles and Practice, 2nd ed. New York: Churchill Livingstone, 1995:710–729.

Chapter 5

Anemia with a Normal MCV and Inappropriately Low Reticulocyte Index

Such anemias are among the most common seen in medicine. Before considering possible etiologies and embarking on a diagnostic workup, make sure that:

1. The HCT/Hgb is reproducibly low. Know the normal levels for your laboratory. In some laboratories an HCT of 34% in a woman is normal. Recognize the variation in normals based on sex, age, and pregnancy.
2. Volume overload is not the etiology (p. 1).

ANEMIA OF RENAL FAILURE
Mechanism

The most important mechanism is decreased marrow erythropoiesis. Decreased marrow red cell production is secondary to decreased **erythropoietin** production and interference with erythropoietic activity by uremic toxins. In addition, evidence suggests that excessive parathormone activity may inhibit erythropoiesis by causing marrow fibrosis in some patients with renal failure and secondary hyperparathyroidism. A hemolytic component is present as well in severe renal insufficiency, but it is usually mild and one for which a normal marrow production would

Table 5.1
Anemia with a Normal MCV and Low Reticulocyte Index

Differential Diagnosis

Renal failure
Anemia of chronic disease (infection, inflammation, malignancy)
Anemia of hypoendocrine states (hypothyroidism, etc.)
Mild (early) iron deficiency
Combined microcytic and macrocytic anemia
Sideroblastic anemia
Primary bone marrow disorders (aplastic anemia, leukemia, myeloma, etc.)
Bone marrow infiltration (myelophthisis)

compensate. A patient may occasionally develop splenomegaly and severe hemolysis. Be aware that patients on chronic dialysis have other mechanisms for anemia:

- **Iron deficiency** (bleeding into the coil, phlebotomies, GI bleeding)
- **Folate deficiency** (folic acid is hemodialyzable).
- **Microangiopathic hemolysis** (some patients with glomerulopathies, hemolytic uremic syndrome).

Routine Database

The RBC morphology is usually normal. One may see occasional spiculated cells ("burr cells") and schistocytes. An occasional patient may have a microangiopathic smear. Polymorphonuclear leukocytes may be hypersegmented in the absence of folate deficiency. Mild thrombocytopenia (90,000–140,000) is not unusual in severe renal insufficiency. The degree of anemia varies in general with the degree of renal insufficiency. Anemia is usually seen with creatinine clearances less than 20. The HCT level in the absence of erythropoietin treatment is quite variable (low teens with a transfusion requirement to the low 30s).

Additional Database

- **Serum Ferritin**
    An inadequate iron supply is common in renal failure and the most common cause of inadequate erythropoietin responses.

Serum ferritins less than 50 ng/ml should be considered indicative of iron deficiency. Ferritin should be monitored in patients on erythropoietin and kept >50 ng/ml.
- **Serum iron (SI) and total iron-binding capacity (TIBC)**
    Transferrin saturation should be kept >30% in patients on erythropoietin.

Treatment

Dialysis patients are benefitted by the following:

- Supplemental iron and folate administration
- Limit blood drawing.
- Peritoneal dialysis patients have higher hematocrits than hemodialysis patients (more effective in removing those toxins which depress erythropoiesis).
- **Erythropoietin** administration. The majority of dialysis and nondialysis patients with renal failure will respond (max response in around 10 weeks) to 50–100 u/kg given 3 times a week (IV or subcutaneous). Objective is HCTs of 32–38%. Refractoriness is usually due to iron deficiency (rarely aluminum toxicity or secondary hyperparathyroidism). A small percentage of patients will require higher doses of erythropoietin (watch out for hypertension). An extra benefit of elevation of the hematocrit is improvement of the bleeding time (p. 104).

ANEMIA OF CHRONIC DISEASE
Clinical Setting

This is one of the most common mechanisms of anemia and is seen in the setting of almost any chronic inflammatory state (including infections and metastatic malignancy). This anemia has been best studied in rheumatoid arthritis but may be seen in chronic infections, chronic inflammatory liver disease, chronic inflammatory joint disease other than rheumatoid (inflammatory osteoarthritis, gout, etc.), active collagen vascular disease, etc. The mechanism of anemia seen commonly in cancer patients is similar. In addition to these chronic conditions anemia may also develop during acute infections or inflammation of other types.

Mechanism

The major effect is decreased RBC production, although there is also a slight shortening of RBC survival. Decreased production is secondary to inadequate **erythropoietin** release, inhibition of erythropoietin action, and an alteration in **iron kinetics.** Activation of macrophages and lymphocytes secondary to cellular damage leads to sequestration of iron in macrophages, some shortening of red cell survival, and the release of **cytokines** (mainly **interleukin-1** [IL-1], **tumor necrosis factor-alpha** [TNF], and **interferon**) leading to inadequate erythropoietin levels and function. Also, **lactoferrin** released from granulocytes competes with transferrin for iron and contributes to increased macrophage trapping of iron. This decrease in iron availability may have some utility in fighting infections with iron requiring organisms.

Routine Database

The RBC morphology is normal. The MCV is usually normal but may be less than 80 fl. Hypochromia (MCHC <31) is more common that microcytosis. The anemia is mild to moderate. This mechanism does not explain an HCT of less than 25%.

Additional Database Information

The **SI** is low and, if the anemia is chronic, the **TIBC** is low as well. The percent saturation may be as low as 10% but is usually higher than the saturations seen in severe chronic iron deficiency (where the TIBC is frequently elevated). The serum ferritin is normal or elevated, and bone marrow iron stores are normal or increased (increased macrophage iron but absent in red cell precursors [sideroblasts]). As with chronic renal failure, the **serum ferritin** can be used to diagnose iron deficiency in patients with chronic inflammatory states; however, the lower limit of normal should be raised (perhaps 60 ng/ml). A number of malignancies are associated with very elevated serum ferritin levels (p. 14).

Remember:

- Acute infections (viral, bacterial, etc.) may cause an immediate decrease in marrow production, reticulocytopenia and a drop in the SI (within 24 hours). If present for 1–2 weeks, an HCT drop of several percentage points may occur.
- Acute infections (or inflammation of other types) may inhibit the normal bone marrow response to any anemia (bleeding, hemolysis, etc.).

Treatment

It is important to attempt to rule out the simultaneous presence of iron deficiency (common in rheumatic states where nonsteroidal drugs are frequently used), but this may be difficult to do because of the alterations in the usual tests for iron deficiency. Be suspicious, especially in the setting of nonsteroidal use, of ferritins less than 100 ng/ml, and major drops in MCV from the baseline. Empiric trials of iron may be indicated.

Many patients will respond to **erythropoietin.** Best studied are patients with AIDS, rheumatoid arthritis, cancer, and multiple myeloma. Recommended starting doses are 100–150 u/kg, given 3 times a week. The more severe the anemia and the lower the baseline erythropoietin levels the better the response. Good clinical judgment and restraint should be used in deciding the appropriateness of using expensive treatment for mild anemias.

ANEMIA OF HYPOENDOCRINE STATES
Mechanism

The **anemia of hypothyroidism** is best studied. However, anemia also occurs in hypoadrenalism and hypopituitarism. The chief mechanism appears to be decreased red cell production secondary to decreased erythropoietin production probably related to lessened peripheral oxygen requirements. **Other mechanisms** for anemia are common in patients with hypothyroidism:

1. Increased incidence of **pernicious anemia.**
2. **Folic acid deficiency** secondary to decreased intake and possibly malabsorption of folate.
3. **Iron deficiency** (women because of menorrhagia)

Routine Database

The anemia is usually mild (HCTs in low 30s, rarely <25%). The MCV is normal or high normal. A macrocytic anemia in hypothyroidism (MCV >100) is usually due to **pernicious anemia.** The MCV in the anemia of hypothyroidism frequently falls slowly with treatment but is usually not >100. RBCs on smear appear normal. In up to 30% of patients one may find occasional bluntly **spiculated cells.**

Additional Database

Studies for B_{12} deficiency and iron deficiency are appropriate when the routine database suggests these diagnoses. A high percentage of patients have antibodies to parietal cells and intrinsic factor. Gastric achlorhydria is common.

Treatment

In the anemia of hypothyroidism, thyroid replacement results in a slow rise in the hematocrit that may not normalize for many months.

MILD IRON DEFICIENCY

Iron deficiency is discussed in Chapter 2. Remember that the MCV and peripheral smear RBC morphology are usually normal in early, mild iron deficiency anemia. The serum ferritin and bone marrow iron stain will be the most helpful diagnostic tests in such cases. In very early iron deficiency anemia the serum ferritin may be in the low normal range at a time when the bone marrow reveals absent iron stores.

COMBINED IRON DEFICIENCY AND MEGALOBLASTIC ANEMIA

It is not uncommon to see iron deficiency and folate deficiency occurring together in the alcoholic patient or the patient with severe inflammatory small bowel disease. Iron deficiency is also seen sometimes in association with pernicious anemia.

Routine Database

The MCV may be normal, high or low. The smear may show macroovalocytes as well as small hypochromic cells, but the smear may be relatively unhelpful in distinguishing combined deficiency from megaloblastic anemia alone.

Additional Database

Usual diagnostic tests for iron deficiency and folate/B_{12} deficiency.

SIDEROBLASTIC ANEMIA

Sideroblastic anemia is a syndrome with many different etiologies associated with the presence of **ringed sideroblasts** seen on a bone marrow iron stain.

Sideroblastic Anemia: Differential Diagnosis

Congenital
Acquired
    Primary idiopathic
    Secondary
        Drugs (alcohol, lead, antituberculotic drugs, chloramphenicol)
        Collagen vascular disease
        Multiple myeloma
        Marked hemolysis
        Thalassemia
        Megaloblastic anemia
        Myelodysplasia and the nonlymphocytic acute leukemias

The mechanism has been best worked out in the congenital and drug-induced cases. Inhibition of heme metabolism within the mitochrondria is associated with iron loading of the nucleated RBC mitochrondria which are situated in a perinuclear location, resulting in the morphologic picture seen on iron staining of nucleated RBCs (ringed sideroblasts). Alcohol is by far the most common etiology and is frequently seen associated with folate-deficient megaloblastosis. The acquired idiopathic form (**myelodysplastic syndrome,** p. 24) manifests itself as a refractory anemia seen in elderly patients and the MCV is frequently mildly elevated. Some of these patients progress to develop acute non-lymphocytic leukemia, sometimes after many years.

Routine Database

In the congenital and primary idiopathic forms of the disease there is usually marked anisocytosis and poikilocytosis. There is frequently a population of hypochromic, microcytic cells, giving the appearance of two populations of cells. The **MCV,** however, is usually normal or slightly **elevated.** It may on occasion be decreased (congenital forms). Coarse stippling (Pappenheimer bodies) is almost always present but may require a tedious search to find. The bone marrow picture varies with etiology but usually shows erythroid hyperplasia. Iron stain reveals the presence of ringed sideroblasts (nucleated RBCs staining heavily from iron located in the perinuclear mitochrondria).

Additional Database

The **SI** is frequently elevated. The **serum ferritin** is high. Other data will vary depending on etiology. The primary idiopathic and preleukemic forms of the disease may mimic megaloblastic anemia, but the serum B_{12} and serum folate levels are normal or elevated and there is no response to B_{12} or folic acid.

Treatment

Treatment depends on etiology:

- Alcohol—alcohol withdrawal/folic acid administration
- Megaloblastic anemia—late/B_{12}
- Drug induced—(g withdrawal), chelation treatment for lead
- **Primary idiopathic acquired**—Pyridoxine in 200 mg/day doses and folic acid are tried initially and ineffective. Androgens may occasionally delay the time to transfusion requirement. When the hematocrit allows, phlebotomy to remove iron from mitochondria may occasionally be effective as may chelation with **desferrioxamine.** There is a low response rate to **erythropoietin,** which is enhanced with the addition of granulocyte or granulocyte/macrophage **colony stimulating factor. Transfusion** support becomes necessary at some point and iron chelation therapy should then be considered.

APLASTIC ANEMIA

Chronic aplastic anemia will not be described in detail. Severe cases require specialized treatment in a center equipped for bone marrow transplantation. The red cells usually appear normal or demonstrate moderate anisocytosis. The MCV may be normal or slightly elevated. There is a peripheral pancytopenia which may be marked, and the bone marrow is significantly hypocellular. Note that chemotherapy-induced aplasia [azathioprine (Imuran), 6-mercaptopurine, methotrexate, hydroxyurea, 5-fluorouracil, cytosine arabinoside, etc.] often results in a macrocytic peripheral RBC population with morphologic changes of a megaloblastic anemia.

ANEMIA ASSOCIATED WITH BONE MARROW INFILTRATION

Marrow infiltration from various causes is usually associated with a normocytic (occasionally macrocytic) anemia. When infiltration is extensive, there may be classic peripheral blood findings present. These findings, known as **leukoerythroblastosis,** include:

1. Marked variation in red cell shape, "tear drop" cells are common.
2. Nucleated RBCs.
3. Left shift in the granulocytes with myelocytes (or earlier precursors being seen on smear.)

Apparently the disrupted marrow releases cells early. Inappropriately released red cells, still containing cytoplasmic and nuclear fragments, are distorted during passage through the circulation, producing the poikilocytosis.

Leukoerythroblastosis (common etiologies)
Primary myelofibrosis (agnogenic myeloid metaplasia)
End-stage polycythemia vera
Extensive cancer metastases to bone marrow
    Breast
    Prostate
    Oat cell lung cancer
Acute leukemia
Other hematologic malignancies on occasion [chronic lymphocytic leukemia (CLL), multiple myeloma, lymphosarcoma]

Other (miliary tuberculosis, Gaucher's disease, granulomatous disorders)

Leukoerythroblastosis is not a sensitive indicator of bone marrow involvement in metastatic cancer. It is present in less than 25% of cases with a positive bone marrow biopsy for tumor. Anemia is present in most cases with positive bone marrow biopsies.

ANEMIA IN THE ELDERLY

Old age is not an explanation for a significant normocytic anemia. Average hematocrits in patients in their 70s and 80s are only 1–2 percentage points lower than the normal general adult range. However, there are data to suggest that the incidence of unexplained mild anemias increases with age. The issue is difficult to study, given the frequent occurrence of occult disease in the elderly. "Mild anemia of aging" should be a diagnosis of exclusion.

DIAGNOSTIC HELP IN NORMOCYTIC ANEMIAS
The Peripheral Smear

Peripheral RBC morphology confirms the lack of appropriate bone marrow response in normocytic anemias (no polychromatophilia). Some of these conditions are associated with abnormal and specific RBC morphologic abnormalities (Table 5.2).

Table 5.2
Help from the Peripheral Smear

Normal RBC Morphology
   Anemia of chronic disease (malignancy)
   Chronic renal failure (most patients)
   Hypoendocrine states (most patients)
   Early iron deficiency
   Aplastic anemia
Abnormal RBC Morphology
   Combined iron and folate deficiency
   Sideroblastic anemia
   Leukoerythroblastosis
   Renal failure (some patients)
   Hypothyroidism (some patients)

Table 5.3
Help from the Bone Marrow

Bone Marrow Not Helpful:
  Anemia of chronic disease
  Chronic renal failure
  Hypoendocrine states
Bone Marrow Helpful:
  Myelophthisis (marrow biopsy)
  Mild iron deficiency (serum ferritin is cheaper and less uncomfortable)
  Combined iron deficiency and megaloblastic anemia
  Sideroblastic anemia
  Aplastic anemia
  Primary marrow malignancy (leukemia, myeloma, etc.)
  Marrow infiltration

Indications for a Bone Marrow Examination

In general the bone marrow offers minimal help in the workup of the most common of these anemias and should not be obtained routinely (Table 5.3).

THE PATIENT WITH CHRONIC, VERY MILD ANEMIA AND NO OBVIOUS CAUSE

One of the most frustrating problems encountered by the primary physician is that of a very mild anemia (**HCT 35 in a woman or 40 in a man**) with a normal MCV, smear, reticulocyte count, and no clues regarding etiology from the problem list. Consider the following explanations:

1. Fluid overload
2. Recent considerable blood loss from phlebotomy during hospitalization, especially in the setting of a febrile illness inhibiting bone marrow response
3. Recent inflammatory problem (including viral infection, recent myocardial infarction, etc.)
4. 2.5% of a normal population will have a hematocrit lower than the lower limit of normal.
5. Hematocrits from patients are lower when supine compared to when sitting (increase in plasma volume).

Recommendations

1. Consider the differential diagnosis listed earlier in the chapter and the comments above.

2. If none seem likely or pertinent, and the anemia has just been recognized (especially during a recent hospitalization), it is reasonable to follow the HCT in the outpatient setting without further diagnostic workup while realizing the presence of an unexplained problem.

3. If it is known that the anemia is relatively recent (e.g., normal HCT 3 months ago), it should be explained. Consider first:
   a. Occult GI bleeding and early iron deficiency anemia.
   b. Anemia of chronic disease/malignancy (recent weight loss, fever, etc?).

4. Hypothyroidism. It is often unsuspected and undiagnosed until present for months to years.

Suggested Reading

Erslev AJ. Anemia of chronic disease. In: Beutler E, Lichtman MA, Coller BS, Kipps TJ, eds. Williams: Hematology. New York: McGraw-Hill, 1995:518–528.

Erslev AJ. Anemia of chronic renal failure. In: Beutler E, Lichtman MA, Coller BS, Kipps TJ, eds. Williams: Hematology. New York: McGraw-Hill, 1995:456–462.

Erslev AJ. Anemia of hypoendocrine states. In: Beutler E, Lichtman MA, Coller BS, Kipps TJ, eds. Williams: Hematology. New York: McGraw-Hill, 1995:462–466.

Lipochitz DA, Udupa KB, Milton KY, Thompson CO. Effect of age on hematopoiesis in man. Blood 1984;63:502–509.

Means RT, Krantz SB. Progress in understanding the pathogenesis of the anemia of chronic disease. Blood 1992;80:1639.

Wiley JS. Sideroblastic anemias. In: Hoffman R, Benz EJ, Shattil SJ, Furie B, Cohen HJ, Silberstein LE, eds. Hematology: Basic Principles and Practice. New York: Churchill Livingstone, 1995:545–552.

Chapter 6

Hemoglobin S and Hemoglobin C Disorders

Congenital disorders of globin chain synthesis may cause several different clinical syndromes:

- Hemolysis (unstable hemoglobins, e.g., Hgb Zurich)
- Erythrocytosis (increased Hgb O_2 affinity, e.g., Hgb Chesapeake)
- Cyanosis (e.g., Hgb Kansas and Hgb Seattle)

The above syndromes are quite rare in comparison with hemoglobin S and hemoglobin C disorders.

HEMOGLOBIN S

- Hemoglobin S is a β chain mutation resulting in a hemoglobin molecule that aggregates with deoxygenation and hypertonic milieus forming rigid fibers of hemoglobin S that distort cell shape and damage cell membranes. Membrane damage leads to potassium and intracellular fluid loss and a marked increase in cellular hemoglobin concentration (MCHC). This intracellular hypertonicity further stimulates sickle hemoglobin polymerization resulting ultimately in dense, irreversibly sickled cells that have a short survival, adhere to vascular endothelial cell membranes, and ultimately occlude vessels.
- Eight percent of the African American population in the United States is heterozygous for Hgb S (Hgb AS).

- The gene is also present to a lesser extent in Greeks, Italians, Arabians and Asian Indians.
- The mutation affords protection from endemic malaria.

Sickle Cell Trait (Hgb AS)

- For the most part, sickle trait individuals are completely well, although many rare clinical problems have been associated with the sickle cell trait defect. Those for which there are reasonable data to support a cause-effect relationship are:

  1. Splenic infarction at high altitudes.
  2. Episodic hematuria.
  3. Increased incidence of bacteriuria including bacteriuria and pyelonephritis in pregnancy.
  4. Hyposthenuria.
  5. Unexplained sudden death with very strenuous exercise (rare).

Many other anecdotal associations are much less well documented.

- **The peripheral smear is normal.** Sickling is seen only on a sickle cell prep (deoxygenated blood).
- **Hemoglobin electrophoresis** reveals 25–40% Hgb S and the rest Hgb A, with a small amount of Hgb F and Hgb A_2.
- Once identified, sickle cell trait individuals should receive:

  1. **Genetic counseling**
     a. Information about the incidence of Hgb S gene.
     b. A couple, both heterozygous for Hgb S, have a 25% chance of having a child with sickle cell anemia. A couple has a 25% chance of having a child with hemoglobin SC disease or hemoglobin S-β-thalassemia when one is heterozygous for hemoglobin S and the other heterozygous for hemoglobin C or β-Thalassemia.
  2. Assurance that they are essentially clinically normal, and that complications from carrying the sickle cell gene are extremely rare.

Sickle Cell Anemia (Hgb SS)

Hemoglobin SS disease exists in approximately 0.25% of the African American population in the United States. Clinical sequelae of this serious disease differ in pediatric and adult populations. The pediatrician primarily sees infectious complications related to decreased bacterial opsonization, decreased reticuloendothelial system (RES) phagocytosis and possibly increased bacterial load from gastrointestinal (GI) ischemia. Pneumococcal and haemophilus infections predominate. Salmonella osteomyelitis is also common. The physician caring for adults primarily sees organ dysfunction complications, the result of repeated ischemic events in various body organs. Both commonly see painful sickle cell crises.

General Laboratory Findings

Anemia. Normocytic or slightly macrocytic because of the reticulocytosis. Hct ranges from high teens to low 30s. The mechanism is primarily hemolytic, and a chronic indirect hyperbilirubinemia is common. Although some cells are dehydrated appearing hyperchromic, the MCHC is usually normal (increased in SC disease).

Leukocytosis. There may be a chronic neutrophilia, and WBC counts may rise to 30,000–40,000/µl with pain crises.

Thrombocytosis. Usually mild. May be greater than 1,000,000/µl.

Reticulocytosis.

Peripheral smear. Markedly distorted red cell shapes with classic sickled erythrocytes evident on a routine smear. Polychromatophilia is prominent. **Howell-Jolly bodies** and **Pappenheimer bodies** are common features of autosplenectomy from sickling (usually occurring before age 10). Target cells are usual (most prominent in SC disease).

Hgb electrophoresis. Reveals only Hgb S with a variable amount of Hgb F (no Hgb A).

Effect on Various Organ Systems

Bone. There are a number of clinical and radiologic features commonly seen in sickle cell bone disease:

- Widened medullary spaces in the proximal long bones and skull due to significant compensatory bone marrow expansion.
- **"Codfish" spine:** Central circumscribed areas of depression in the vertebral end plates.

- Ischemia and infarction leading to **changes that mimic osteomyelitis** (periosteal reaction, osteosclerosis, etc.). Osteomyelitis is common as well.
- **Dactylitis (hand-foot syndrome).** Acute swelling of hands and feet seen in infants.
- **Aseptic necrosis** of the femoral (and rarely humoral) head (more common in Hgb SC disease).
- **Bone marrow necrosis** sometimes with bone marrow embolization.
- Growth is inhibited. Children are short and puberty is delayed, and many adult sickle cell patients are tall with long thin extremities.

Spleen. Splenomegaly disappears usually by age 8 as a result of repeated infarctions. This autosplenectomy state contributes to the tendency to infection and causes some peripheral blood changes noted above. Splenic sequestration crisis occurs in infants because of massive splenic pooling of red cells and is frequently fatal. Adults with hemoglobin SC and S-b-thalassemia frequently have functional and enlarged spleens.

Liver and Gallbladder. Hepatomegaly may occur with crises. Pain crises mimic acute cholecystitis or other abdominal catastrophes.

Intrahepatic cholestasis secondary to sickling in the sinusoids may occur, resulting in massive hyperbilirubinemia (combination of hemolysis and hepatic dysfunction), with bilirubin levels sometimes greater than 100 mg%).

Differentiation of the above syndromes from cholecystitis is difficult (50% of adult sickle cell patients have **gallstones,** about 50% of which are radio opaque bilirubin stones). Indications for cholecystectomy are not distinct. Many physicians recommend elective **cholecystectomy** in sickle cell patients with gallstones who have had abdominal episodes consistent with acute cholecystitis. Several large series have demonstrated that elective cholecystectomy is relatively safe in SS patients.

Cardiovascular. Patients develop cardiomegaly from chronic anemia and repetitive microinfarctions. Murmurs are frequent and may suggest rheumatic or congenital heart disease.

Pulmonary. The **acute chest syndrome** is common in sickle cell patients. The syndrome is characterized by fever, chest pain, pronounced leukocytosis, and pulmonary infiltrates on chest x-ray. The etiology is infection or thrombosis/embolism and it is usually difficult to distinguish which one clinically (rib infarction may also play a role in some cases). Severity varies considerably and death may occur, especially in children. Treatment is controversial. Antibiotics and supportive treatment are usually given; exchange transfusion is reserved for more seriously ill patients. Deep venous thrombosis and pulmonary embolism occur in sickle patients and should be treated with standard anticoagulation therapy. Pulmonary thrombosis/embolism may be extensive and recurrent and lead, with time, to pulmonary hypertension and right heart failure.

Central Nervous System. Vascular accidents are common, especially in children under the age of 15, and include cerebral infarction, cerebral hematomas, and subdural and subarachnoid hemorrhage. Seizure disorders are seen frequently and recurrence is quite common (65% within 3 years of the original event). Persuasive evidence demonstrates that a program of hypertransfusion, to decrease Hgb S percent, following a CNS vascular event is useful in preventing recurrence. Exchange transfusion seems to be helpful in decreasing the chance of complications of **arteriography** (high in sickle cell disease).

Leg Ulcers. Up to 75% of patients with SS disease develop leg ulcerations at some time during their lives, and for many the problem is chronic. The following are characteristic features:

- Usually seen on the medial side of the leg above the ankle.
- Typically presents a punched-out appearance and may be quite large.
- Thought to be due to ischemia in an area where venous pressure is high.
- Many treatments have been tried. No clear evidence exists of increased benefit of one compared with another.

Eye. Sickle cell patients, including patients with SC and S-b-thalassemia. disease, are prone to retinopathy, which, although potentially preventable, may lead to blindness. The following patho-physiologic sequence occurs:

1. Retinal capillary plugging by sickled cells.
2. Secondary **neovascularization** (arborization) resulting in fragile vascular connections between arterioles and venules. They are located at the periphery of the retinas and look like a primitive marine animal known as a sea fan.
3. **Vitreous hemorrhage** secondary to leak in one of these defective vessels.
4. Retinal detachment as the vitreous hemorrhage scars and retracts.

The above sequence can be interrupted prior to the vitreous hemorrhage by laser coagulation of the abnormal new vessels. Every patient with SS, SC and S-thalassemia disease should have a yearly evaluation by an ophthalmologist with experience in these techniques.

Kidney. SS (SA, SC, S-β-thalassemia) patients have hyposthenuria and may develop episodes of severe unilateral hematuria secondary to ischemia of the renal medulla. In addition to renal tubular dysfunction, immune complex glomerular disease is sometimes seen.

OTHER SICKLE CELL SYNDROMES

SC Disease

Slightly milder than SS disease. Smear reveals many target cells common with all C hemoglobinopathies. The Hgb electrophoresis reveals approximately equal levels of Hgb C and Hgb S. The spleen may be palpable.

S-β-Thalassemia

Slightly milder than SS disease. The MCV is low. Target cells may be prominent on smear. The spleen may be palpable. Hgb electrophoresis reveals a pattern of 70–80% S with small amounts of Hgb A and F. In S-β_0-thalassemia there is no hemoglobin A present; hemoglobin A_2 may be elevated.

S-α-Thalassemia

Coexistent α-thalassemia occurs in approximately $\frac{1}{3}$ of sickle cell patients ($\frac{1}{3}$ American blacks have alpha thalassemia). Patients with sickle cell α- thalassemia have higher hematocrits and lower MCVs. Thalassemic red cells have redundant membranes which allow more cell stretching before damage. Compared to SS cells, SS-α thalassemia cells lose less potassium during intracellular sickling and thus become less dehydrated. By becoming less dense (maintaining a lower MCHC) during deoxygenation, irreversible sickling is prevented and cell viability is favored. However, the high hematocrit seen in SS-α thalassemia results in an increased viscosity, and there is some evidence suggesting increased incidence of retinal damage and osteonecrosis.

C-Trait Disease (Hgb AC)

Present in 2–3% of American blacks. Usually clinically normal without anemia. The smear reveals large numbers of target cells.

Hgb CC Disease

A mild disease associated with a slight anemia, splenomegaly and occasional mild pain (arthralgia). Infections may be seen, including Salmonella osteomyelitis. The smear reveals target cells and misshapen spherocytes (common in all the C hemoglobinopathies), as well as dense intracellular hemoglobin crystals.

Hgb SS with High Hgb F

Elevated hemoglobin F levels are clinically beneficial in sickle cell disease as demonstrated by the mild disease seen in the Arabian form of Sickle Cell anemia and by patients doubly heterozygous for Hgb S and hereditary persistence of hemoglobin F. Hgb F interrupts Hgb S polymerization and protects against intracellular sickling. Levels greater than 10% appear to protect against strokes and osteonecrosis, and levels greater than 20% protect against painful crises.

TREATMENT
Pain (Thrombotic) Crisis

Pain may involve any area of the body, but commonly involves long bones, the back and the abdomen. The pain is frequently severe, requiring parenteral narcotics. Crises may last a few hours to days and even, rarely, several weeks. The patient may have fever (occasionally to 104°) and an increase in the usual neutrophilia, making differentiation from infection difficult. Hospitalization with appropriate narcotics for pain control is often necessary; however, there is no specific treatment. Data do not support the helpfulness of nasal oxygen in the absence of significant hypoxia. It is reasonable to maintain good hydration; inability to concentrate the urine contributes to dehydration during febrile illnesses. The most important medical issue is to rule out infection. The patient must be tapered off narcotics before discharge as iatrogenic addiction does occur.

Infection

As mentioned, these patients, especially children, are very prone to infections (pneumococcal, Haemophilus, Salmonella), and should be encouraged to see their physicians early for any febrile illness. Because of the sickle-cell patient's difficulty with handling pneumococcal infections, it is recommended that he or she be immunized with pneumococcal vaccine. Children are given prophylactic penicillin until the age of 6.

Hemolytic Crisis

Such crises are rare in adults where a hematocrit drop occurring in the setting of a pain crisis should make the physician suspect infection. Infection decreases marrow red cell production resulting in a rapid hematocrit drop in the severe, chronic hemolytic anemia patient.

Aplastic Crisis

Decreased marrow production results in a dramatic hematocrit drop in these patients. Infection is the most common etiology. A **pure red cell aplasia** occurs with **parvovirus infections** and the hematocrit drops dramatically. Transfusions are necessary to support the patient through an otherwise typical acute viral illness. In addition to infection, **folic acid** deficiency may develop because of the patient's increased requirements (marked erythroid hyperplasia) resulting in severe anemia. It is reasonable to maintain sickle cell patients on 1 mg per day of supplemental folic acid.

Thrombosis/Embolization

As with any other patient, sickle cell patients with a deep vein thrombosis or pulmonary embolism should be anticoagulated. Pulmonary thrombosis in situ may develop and may be difficult to distinguish from pneumonia in a febrile patient with leukocytosis.

Leg Ulcers

Ulcers, when large, are particularly refractory to treatment. Skin grafting is helpful in only a minority of patients and often not worth the time and discomfort involved. Local measures to keep the ulcer clean, regular elevation, surgical stockings, and wraps are useful. Frequently healing occurs over months only to recur again a few months or years later.

Hematuria

Common in patients with Hgb AS as well as SS, SC and S-β-thalassemia, it is thought to be caused by medullary ischemia, owing to the tendency of cells to sickle when subjected to the hypertonic milieu of the renal medulla. Bleeding may occur for days to weeks. Maintaining a high urine flow is usually successful in stopping the hematuria.

Priapism

Recurrent priapism is common in SS and SC disease patients and may result in permanent impotence, especially in older adolescents and adults. Urologic intervention may be attempted within the first few hours of onset, but it is not clear that operative intervention is helpful in preventing impotence. Urologic prostheses, once impotence has occurred, are helpful.

PREVENTIVE MEDICINE RECOMMENDATIONS

1. The sickle cell patient has a lifelong illness requiring recurrent use of the medical care system. He or she needs:
   a. **One personal physician.**
   b. **Access** to a physician 24 hours a day.
   c. A workable system to obtain **emergency care** 24 hours a day.
2. **Folic acid** (1 mg per day).
3. Rapid medical evaluation for the development of **fever/ chills.**
4. **Pneumococcal vaccine.**
5. **Analgesics.** Narcotic addiction does occur. In general, the sickle cell patient should probably not be given oral narcotics for use at home during a pain crisis except in the following situation:

   There is one personal physician who knows that he or she is the only physician writing narcotic prescriptions for the patient. In a patient with frequent pain crises, it is reasonable to allow the patient a few narcotic analgesic tablets to be used early during a pain attack in the hope of preventing the necessity of an emergency room visit and hospitalization.
6. **Transfusion** and **exchange transfusion therapy.** In general, transfusions should be avoided because of the hazard of iron overload. Exchange transfusion can interrupt long-persistent pain crises, may be helpful in the patient with severe acute chest syndrome, and may be useful prior to general anesthesia to decrease the chance of hypoxemia-induced sickling. The necessity of exchange transfusion or simple transfusion prior to anesthesia remains unproven as does the prophylactic use of transfusions in pregnancy. Chronic hypertransfusion can decrease the number of crises in patients with incapacity from chronic recurrent episodes of pain, and hypertransfusion is useful in preventing recurrent CNS vascular events.
7. Pharmacologic attempts to **increase hemoglobin F** production hold considerable interest. A recent controlled study reported that hydroxyurea increased hemoglobin F levels and

decreased the number of pain crises in sickle cell patients. Candidates for hydroxyurea therapy need to be carefully selected as the clinical benefits are modest, and long-term side effects are cause for concern.

8. **Bone marrow transplantation** has been carried out on a limited number of sickle cell patients with some encouraging results (ongoing, 22-center national trial for patients less than 16 with severe sickle cell morbidity). Transplant mortality for a disease associated with long survival will continue to limit more widespread use for the present.

Suggested Reading

Beutler E. The sickle cell disorders and related disorders. In: Beutler E, Lichtman MA, Coller BS, Kipps TJ, eds. Williams: Hematology. New York, McGraw-Hill, 1995:616–650.

Brookoff D, Polomano R. Treating sickle cell pain like cancer pain. Ann Intern Med 1992;116:364.

Dover G, Charache S. Hydroxyurea induction of fetal hemoglobin synthesis in sickle-cell disease. Seminars in Oncology, 1992;19:61.

Steinberg MH, Emburg SH. Thalassemia in Blacks: genetic and clinical aspects and interactions with the sickle hemoglobin gene. Blood 1986;68:985–990.

Wayne AS, Kevy SV, Nathan DG. Transfusion management of sickle cell disease. Blood 1993;81:1109.

Chapter 7

Bleeding Disorders: Approach to Diagnosis

DIAGNOSTIC APPROACH TO BLEEDING

When faced with a bleeding patient or a history of untoward bleeding, the clinician should initially try to answer the following clinical questions:

1. Is the Bleeding from More than One Site?

Bleeding from only one site is usually not due to a bleeding diathesis. Beware of the untied bleeder in the operative wound or the recurrent unilateral nosebleed.

2. Is the Bleeding Problem Lifelong or of Recent Onset?

Hereditary bleeding problems are usually easily identified by a history of lifelong bleeding. A family history of bleeding may suggest a pattern of inheritance. However, be wary of the general statement, "I've always been a free bleeder." Apply much greater weight to objective data. For example:

    a. Untoward bleeding with surgery (e.g., tonsillectomy, tooth extraction) especially if **transfusions** were necessary

    b. Bleeding requiring **hospitalization** or return to the dentist for control of delayed bleeding

3. Does the Pattern of Bleeding Suggest a Clotting Problem or a "Hemostatic Plug" Formation Problem?

    a. Clotting problems (for example, hemophilia)

       (1) Bleeding from large vessels, not capillaries

    (2) Hemarthrosis, large hematomas, large ecchymosis, extensive bleeding with trauma

  b. "Hemostatic plug" (platelet) problems?

    (1) Small vessel (capillary) bleeding—petechiae

    (2) Mucous membrane bleeding (nose, gums, GI tract)

    (3) An "ooze" rather than a "gush"

  c. Some bleeding diatheses are associated with both a clotting and a hemostatic plug formation problem (see Chapter 9).

ROUTINE LABORATORY DATABASE

The following tests are available and used as screening tests in most hospitals and represent reasonable and inexpensive baseline data in the evaluation of all patients with a suspected bleeding diathesis.

1. Prothrombin time (PT)
2. Activated partial thromboplastin time (aPTT)
3. Thrombin time (TT)
4. Peripheral smear
5. Platelet count

    The above tests, using the widely employed Vacutainer system, require one citrate tube (PT, aPTT, TT), one ethylenediaminetetraacetic acid (EDTA) tube (platelet count), and a finger stick peripheral smear. Be careful of the following pitfalls in obtaining the routine data:

1. Citrate tubes usually contain 0.5 cc of anticoagulant to which 4.5 cc's of blood should be added. This ratio is important. Incomplete filling of the tube (e.g., partial loss of vacuum) may result in false results, especially of the aPTT.
2. Coagulation tests should be conducted promptly following drawing of blood. The aPTT in particular may be artificially prolonged by delay in assay.
4. Platelet counts may be conducted after sitting at 4°C for up to 24 hours. The platelet count may be spuriously increased in patients with very high WBC counts (leukemia) or severe RBC poikilocytosis (alteration in shape).

The coagulation process used to be conceptualized as an enzymatic cascade consisting of an intrinsic and extrinsic system. The two systems ended in the activation of Factor X (Xa), which in the presence of Factor V, calcium, and phospholipid (P1), converted prothrombin (Factor II) to thrombin. Thrombin converted fibrinogen to fibrin. Recent developments in the understanding of coagulation have altered this conception and the "enzymatic cascade" idea has undergone considerable revision.

In the revised concept of clot formation, the activation of Factor X and the subsequent conversion of prothrombin to thrombin and fibrinogen to fibrin remains the common pathway of clot formation (Fig.7.1). Activated factor X in the presence of Factor V plus lipid (provided by platelets in vivo) results in the subsequent conversion of prothrombin (Factor II) to thrombin. Thrombin cleaves fibrinogen; the resulting fibrin monomer polymerizes to form a clot which is stabilized by Factor XIII. Ca^{++} is necessary in a number of coagulation steps (as is phospholipid primarily supplied by platelets). Blood is anticoagulated in vitro by the binding of CA^{++} (citrate is usually used for coagulation tests).

The concept of two pathways of Factor X activation, an "intrinsic" and "extrinsic" system, has been modified. In vivo there appears to be little or no role played by activation through an intrinsic system of enzymatic cascade. In vivo hemostasis is initiated

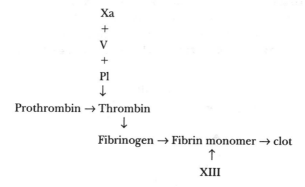

Figure 7.1

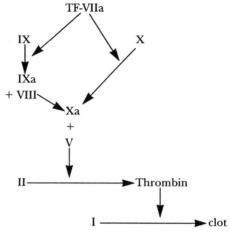

Figure 7.2

through the release of tissue factor (transmembrane glycoprotein present on many cell surfaces). Tissue factor (TF, Factor III) activates Factor VII (VIIa) and the TF-VIIa complex activates Factor X directly. TF-VIIa also activates Factor IX (IXa) which in the presence of Factor VIII and phospholipid also activates Factor X (Fig. 7.2).

Factor X activation results in the release of an inhibitor of TF-VIIa [**Tissue factor pathway inhibitor (TFPI)**]. Thus, continuation of coagulation requires activation of Factor X through the secondary (IXa/VIII) route. Once started the secondary pathway continues without stimulation from TF-VIIa (through stimulation from thrombin generation and perhaps Factor XI). Both methods of ac-

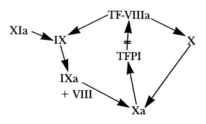

Figure 7.3

tivation of Factor X are necessary for normal hemostasis explaining why hemophiliacs (Factor VIII or Factor IX deficiency) bleed.

Although incorrect in conceptualizing in vivo coagulation, the enzymatic cascade continues to be useful in understanding the common screening tests used in vitro to assess the integrity of the clotting system.

INDIVIDUAL COAGULATION TESTS

Prothrombin Time (PT)

The PT measures primarily Factors II, VII, V and X (Fig.7.4). Calcium plus commercial "thromboplastin," which contains TF plus phospholipid (Pl) provided in vivo by platelets, is added to citrated plasma, and the time to clot formation is measured (11–13 seconds in most systems). The presence of antithrombins (e.g., heparin) or abnormalities in the third stage of coagulation (fibrin generation) will also affect the PT since the formation of a clot is the endpoint of the test. Note that the platelet contribution to coagulation is not measured by the PT as it is a component of the added thromboplastin.

Partial Thromboplastin Time (PTT)

The PTT measures primarily Factors XII, XI, IX, VIII, X and V. (Fig.7.5) Calcium plus phospholipid is added, and the time to

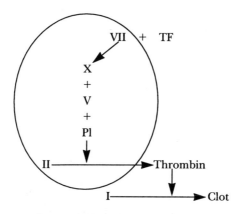

Figure 7.4. Prothrombin time.

clot formation is measured (usually 25–35 seconds in the activated PTT system). The commercial partial thromboplastin added is incapable of activating Factor VII, but provides the phospholipid (Pl) needed in several steps of coagulation (provided in vivo by platelets). As with the PT, subsequent problems in the second and third stages of coagulation will also affect the PTT since the formation of a clot is the endpoint of the test. The PTT also will be prolonged in patients with deficiencies of Factor XII, high-molecular–weight kininogen (HMWK), and prekallikrein (PK), factors not affecting in vivo clotting.

Thrombin Time (TT)

The TT measures only the last stage of coagulation (Fig.7.6). Thrombin and Ca^{++} are added, and the time is measured to form a clot. The TT may be abnormal in the presence of antithrombins (e.g., heparin), with qualitative and quantitative abnormalities of fibrinogen, and when there is a problem with fibrin polymerization.

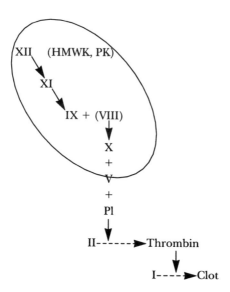

Figure 7.5. Partial thromboplastin time.

Platelet Function

Platelets function to plug small holes in blood vessels. Initially, small numbers of platelets adhere to exposed tissue at the site of a damaged vessel. Platelets release adenosine diphosphate (ADP), which causes large masses of platelets to aggregate ("hemostatic plug" formation), and subsequently release lipid necessary for clot formation. In vitro tests of platelet function require sophisticated equipment and are not part of the routine data base in the evaluation of a bleeding diathesis. The bleeding time is generally not part of the initial routine evaluation of a bleeding diathesis, but it is indicated when the bleeding pattern suggests a hemostatic plug defect with no significant decrease in platelet count.

Peripheral Smear and Platelet Count

The peripheral smear may reveal thrombocytopenia or, rarely, marked thrombocytosis in patients with a bleeding diathesis. In addition, platelet morphology on occasion may be useful. Remember that the smear should be made from a finger stick as anticoagulants distort platelet morphology (swollen, large).

Platelets may distribute unevenly on a smear, so that a "bottle smear" (a smear made from anticoagulated blood) may be better for assessing platelet numbers (the one thing for which a bottle smear may be superior to a finger stick). Red cell morphology on smear may be helpful [for example, as in disseminated intravascular coagulation (DIC) where fragmented red cells (schistocytes) may be seen on smear]. White cell morphology may also be helpful [as when polys reveal the changes associated with sepsis in a patient with DIC (p. 153), or thrombocytopenia associated with sepsis (p. 91)].

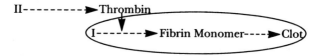

Figure 7.6. Thrombin Time

It is difficult to describe the technique of estimating the platelet count from the peripheral smear, but technicians with considerable experience are quite good at it. The following generalizations may be useful.

1. Platelets are normally present in clumps on smear.
2. Clumps disappear and only single platelets are seen as the count drops to the 100,000/ul range and below.
3. Normally several platelets, some in clumps, are seen in each oil emersion field.
4. Be aware that on a smear platelets may be unequally distributed, located primarily along the sides of the smear.

Suggested Reading

Coller BS, Schneiderman PI. Clinical evaluation of hemorrhagic disorders: bleeding history and differential diagnosis of purpura. In: Hoffman R, Benz EJ, Shattil SJ, Furie B, Cohen HJ, Silberstein LE, eds. Hematology: Basic Principles and Practice. New York: Churchill Livingstone, 1995:1606–1622.

Santoro SA, Eby CS. Laboratory evaluation of hemostatic disorders. In: Hoffman R, Benz EJ, Shattil SJ, Furie B, Cohen HJ, Silberstein LE, eds. Hematology: Basic Principles and Practice. New York: Churchill Livingstone, 1995:1622–1632.

Suchman AC, Griner PF. Diagnostic uses of the activated partial thromboplastin time and prothrombin time. Ann Intern Med 1986;104: 810.

Chapter 8

Disorders of Platelets

THROMBOCYTOPENIA (TABLE 8.1)

As described in Chapter 6, platelets form the major line of defense against bleeding from small holes in blood vessels. This **"hemostatic plug"** function requires adequate platelet numbers as well as normal platelet function.

Platelets made in the bone marrow circulate for approximately 10 days before removal from the circulation. Young platelets are more functional than old platelets.

The normal platelet count, using automatic counters, usually ranges from 150,000 to 350,000/μl. There are technical problems which may yield erroneously low counts (**pseudothrombocytopenia**). The most common cause is the presence of platelet agglutinins in the patient's plasma that cause platelet clumping in vitro (incidence 0.1%). Usually this is seen in EDTA anticoagulated blood. Low counts must be verified by an examination of the smear for platelet clumping and sometimes, when **pseudothrombocytopenia** is suspected, checking the platelet level using another anticoagulant (usually citrate). These agglutinins (antibodies) have no clinical significance and are usually persistent over time. A platelet count, or at least an estimation of platelet numbers on a peripheral smear, is part of the routine database obtained on any patient with a suspected bleeding diathesis. The appropriate routine data to be obtained in patients with thrombocytopenia are listed below:

Routine Data Base (Table 8.2)

- **Platelet count** (with confirmation of thrombocytopenia by examination of a peripheral smear).

Table 8.1
Thrombocytopenia: Differential Diagnosis

Decreased Survival, Sequestration
  Hypersplenism
  TTP/hemolytic uremic syndrome
  DIC
  Sepsis
  Immune thrombocytopenia
Decreased Production
  Myelophthisis
  Primary bone marrow disorders
  Infection
  Drugs (marrow depressant)
Ineffective Production
  Megaloblastic processes

- **History and physical** examination with review of the **problem list** for likely etiologies of thrombocytopenia.
- Examination of **platelet morphology** on a finger stick peripheral smear.
- **Bone marrow examination** (often not necessary).

Etiologic Hints from the Routine Database

Severe thrombocytopenia (platelet counts less than 20,000).
Consider:

1. Immune thrombocytopenia.
2. Severe aplastic anemia (including drug-induced bone marrow depression).
3. Acute leukemia and other primary marrow disorders.

Peripheral smear **platelet morphology**

1. **Young platelets** released in severe thrombocytopenia are large and elongated when seen on a peripheral smear. In severe

Table 8.2
Thrombocytopenia: Routine Database

Mechanism	Platelet Size	Megakaryocyte Numbers
Decreased survival	Large	Increased
Decreased production	Small	Decreased
Ineffective production	Variable	Normal or increased

thrombocytopenia the presence of such platelets suggests a destructive/sequestration mechanism (e.g., immune thrombocytopenia).

2. **Old platelets** are small. A predominance of small platelets on a smear in severe thrombocytopenia suggests a production mechanism (e.g., aplastic anemia). Production thrombocytopenias are sometimes associated with large, morphologically abnormal platelets (Myelodysplasia).

Bone marrow **megakaryocytes**

1. Increased in destructive thrombocytopenia.
2. Decreased in productive thrombocytopenia.
3. Frequently increased in ineffective megakaryocytopoiesis (e.g., in megaloblastic processes). Other bone marrow findings usually help distinguish between a. and c.

On the basis of the above considerations, the physician should attempt to classify the basic mechanism of the thrombocytopenia.

BASIC MECHANISMS

1. Shortened platelet survival or increased peripheral sequestration.
2. Decreased production.
3. Ineffective production.

Shortened Platelet Survival or Increased Sequestration

Normally, platelets survive for about 10 days once released into the circulatory system. Approximately 30% of the circulating platelets are sequestered at any one time in the spleen. Table 8.3

Table 8.3
Destruction/Sequestration Thrombocytopenia: Differential Diagnosis

Hypersplenism
TTP/hemolytic uremic syndrome
DIC
Infection
Immune thrombocytopenia

lists disorders which are associated with decreased survival and/or increased splenic sequestration.

Routine Database

- The platelet count may be mildly or severely decreased. When it is less than 20,000, suspect immune thrombocytopenia.
- Platelet morphology on a smear reveals some large, frequently elongated platelets.
- The bone marrow reveals increased numbers of megakaryocytes.

Hypersplenism

Thrombocytopenia may occur with splenomegaly of almost any etiology, although sometimes it is not present even with massive splenic enlargement. Often leukopenia is present as well. Significant anemia is less common. Approximately 30% of peripheral platelets are contained in the spleen at any given time. In hypersplenism up to 90% of peripheral platelets may be sequestered in the spleen.

Another cause of splenic sequestration of platelets is hypothermia.

Treatment. Thrombocytopenia is rarely severe enough to require splenectomy in hypersplenism. Patients with leukemic reticuloendotheliosis and pancytopenia benefit from splenectomy, as occasionally do patients with chronic lymphocytic leukemia (CLL), lymphomas and myeloproliferative diseases.

Thrombotic Thrombocytopenic Purpura (TTP)/Hemolytic Uremic Syndromes (HUS)

These syndromes are associated with microangiopathic hemolysis with schistocytes (p. 40) seen on peripheral smear. TTP is a syndrome classically presenting with rapid onset of thrombocytopenia and intravascular microangiopathic hemolysis [high lactate dehydrogenase (LDH), hemoglobinuria, and hemosiderinuria (p. 37)] associated with endothelial damage, platelet aggregation in small blood vessels, and ischemia of various organs, especially the central nervous system. HUS is classically seen in young children post infection, but also in adults secondary to various etiologies. The kidney is the main organ of ischemic damage. Plasmapheresis is the treatment of choice for TTP and anecdotally useful in adult HUS.

Disseminated Intravascular Coagulation (DIC)

Thrombocytopenia is always present in acute DIC, but the bone marrow may be able to compensate completely for the shortened platelet survival (platelet count normal) when DIC is chronic (p. 119). Platelets return to normal slowly over days, once the cause for DIC is corrected, as compared to coagulation abnormalities, many of which normalize rapidly.

Sepsis

Patients with septicemia, especially Gram-negative sepsis, may have thrombocytopenia in the absence of other evidence of DIC. Depending on the type of infection, there are many different mechanisms. Endotoxin stimulates monocytes resulting in membrane changes and platelet aggregation on monocytes. Infections (including viral infections) may decrease platelet production as well. Treatment is directed at the underlying infection, not the thrombocytopenia itself. Usually platelet counts are greater than $20,000/\mu l$.

Immune Thrombocytopenia

Antibody-mediated thrombocytopenia occurs in the conditions listed in Table 8.4. Proof of an antibody mechanism in individual cases is difficult (especially in acute immune thrombocytopenia). In vitro testing for **platelet-associated IgG** is widely available and can be helpful to confirm an immunologic mechanism, especially in chronic cases. Although reasonably sensitive, the test lacks specificity, and results of the test are not available initially to influence diagnosis and treatment decisions. Immune thrombocytopenia is usually severe (less than $10,000/\mu l$, and may be

Table 8.4
Immune Thrombocytopenia: Differential Diagnosis

Primary (ITP, 80% of chronic cases)
Secondary
  Acute
    Acute viral infections
    Drugs (quinine, quinidine, sulfonamides, heparin)
    Post-transfusion purpura
  Chronic (20% of chronic cases)
    Collagen vascular disorders (SLE, scleroderma, mixed connective tis-
      sue disorder)
    Lymphoproliferative disorders (CLL, lymphomas, macroglobulinemia,
      Hodgkins disease, Graves disease, Hashimoto's thyroiditis
    Other immunodeficiency states (HIV, myasthenia gravis, rheumatoid
      arthritis, biliary cirrhosis, sarcoidosis, graft vs. host disease)

$<1,000/\mu l$). Acute immune thrombocytopenia is often drug-induced and rapidly clears with drug withdrawal.

Acute Immune Thrombocytopenia. Acute immune thrombocyto-penia secondary to a drug usually requires no specific treatment other than discontinuation of the drug. Platelet counts usually return to normal in a few days. If the thrombocytopenia is severe (less than 10,000), or there is clinical bleeding (marked pe-techiae, nosebleeds, etc.), many physicians recommend a short course of steroids (40–60 mg of prednisone in divided doses with rapid tapering over 10 days to 3 weeks once counts return to normal). There is no proof of benefit over and above discontinua-tion of the drug alone, although it is felt that there is a vascular stabilizing effect of steroids resulting in less clinical bleeding at a given level of thrombocytopenia. The patient should not receive the drug subsequently.

Post-transfusion Purpura. Classically this syndrome occurs in multiparous women who develop severe thrombocytopenia, usu-ally with fever, 5–8 days posttransfusion. CNS bleeding occurs in 10 % of patients and mortality within the first few days is high. The syndrome is caused by sensitization during pregnancy to one of several common platelet-specific antigens present on fetal platelets but lacking in the mother. An anamnestic antibody re-

Table 8.5
Some Drugs Implicated in Acute Immune Thrombocytopenia

Quinine	Chlorthalidone
Quinidine	Dilantin
Sulfonamides	Gold salts
Rifampin	Heparin
Thiazide diuretics	Heroin (adulterant?)
Furosemide	Cocaine (adulterant?)

sponse results when the patient is exposed again to the antigen via transfusion. The mechanism whereby the patient's own platelets are affected by the immune response is poorly understood.

This is a rare but life-threatening event and treatment must be started early. Steroids are administered, although usually ineffective. IV gamma globulin is helpful, as is plasma exchange. Platelets should not be transfused. Recovery may take up to 6 weeks.

Chronic Immune Thrombocytopenia. Idiopathic thrombocytopenic purpura (**ITP**), also referred to as autoimmune thrombocytopenic purpura, (ATP), may occur at any age. The platelet count on presentation may be extremely low ($1000/\mu l$) or only moderately depressed. Classically mild skin and mucous membrane petechiae and small ecchymoses are seen but may be absent if the platelet count is greater than 20,000/ul. Splenomegaly is not present. When the count is less than $30,000/\mu l$ patients are usually initially treated with **steroids** (40–100 mg of prednisone per day in divided doses). Response is seen within 2–3 weeks in 60–70% of patients. Once the platelet count rises to the 100,000 range, tapering of the prednisone may begin. A drop in prednisone to 40 mg per day (10 mg q6h) can usually be accomplished immediately. Subsequent tapering is at a rate of approximately 5 mg per week. Some patients can be tapered off steroids completely without a drop in platelet count. Others will require an ongoing dose of steroid to maintain an adequate platelet count. **Splenectomy** is usually considered when:

1. The initial steroid treatment (2–3 weeks) does not significantly elevate the platelet count.
2. An unacceptable steroid dose (15 mg or more of prednisone per day) is required to maintain the platelet count at greater than 30–50,000.
3. **CNS bleeding** occurs. Historically, emergency splenectomy was the treatment of choice for this life-threatening rare complication of severe immune thrombocytopenia. The overall response rate is higher with emergency splenectomy, and, most importantly, the average time to response is shorter than with steroid treatment. However, IV gamma globulin (see below) usually gives a rapid platelet response without the risks of surgery. Also, platelet transfusions may be more successful after IV gamma globulin treatment.

Splenectomy responses commonly occur within a few days of surgery, sometimes immediately, but if not within 10 days, usually do not occur. Presently, the indications for splenectomy are not clear cut. A syndrome of overwhelming sepsis is rare in adults postsplenectomy, although common in young children in whom splenectomy is contraindicated under the age of 6. The recognition of this rare but often fatal syndrome has made many hematologists slower to recommend splenectomy for their patients. All patients undergoing splenectomy should receive pneumococcal vaccine and probably vaccination against hemophilus influenza type B at least 2 weeks prior to splenectomy. Although splenectomy is usually successful in rapidly raising the platelet count, with time postsplenectomy relapses are common. Splenectomy should generally be done prior to the use of second-line therapies for refractory ITP.

Severe bleeding in ITP is unusual even with chronic severe thrombocytopenia. The overall mortality from bleeding in ITP is low as is the incidence of CNS bleeding. The objective of treatment is not normalization of the platelet count but maintenance of a reasonably safe level of hemostasis without significant treatment-associated morbidity.

Chronic Secondary Immune Thrombocytopenia. (Table 8.4) Chronic secondary immune thrombocytopenia is treated much like ITP but with a major emphasis placed on treatment of the underlying disease. Patients with underlying lymphoproliferative disorders have a refractory thrombocytopenia until the underlying disease is controlled. There is evidence that splenectomy may be less effective in lupus immune thrombocytopenia than in the idiopathic form. One should always be suspicious of the presence of an associated, underlying disease when patients present with what appears to be ITP and, especially in the elderly, one should search for the presence of an underlying lymphoproliferative disease.

Other Treatment Modalities. **Danazol,** an androgen, has been reported to be effective in ITP and has become the second therapeutic intervention after steroids, and sometimes even before splenectomy, of many hematologists. Usually begun at a dose of 200 mg t.i.d. or q.i.d., it is then tapered to the lowest possible maintenance dose (reportedly, a dose as low as 50 mg daily may be effective). It is primarily used to allow a decrease in steroid dose in patients requiring chronic steroid therapy before or after splenectomy. Side effects include nausea, fluid retention, liver function abnormalities, and minimal masculinization in a small per cent of women. Amenorrhea in women with heavy periods secondary to thrombocytopenia can be helpful.

Intravenous gamma globulin is effective in normalizing the platelet count rapidly in patients with severe ITP. The mechanism is thought to involve neutralization of Fc receptors on reticuloendothelial cells primarily in the spleen. The effect is short lived (two weeks on average). Large doses are given by slow intravenous infusion over 2–5 days. The treatment is expensive and indications are not universally agreed on, but include serious bleeding (such as CNS bleeds) or potential for serious bleeding (major surgery). Elective splenectomy in the uncomplicated patient usually does not require intravenous gamma globulin prior to surgery as significant bleeding is unusual.

Anti-Rh(D) has also been used in Rh(D)+ patients to cause mild hemolysis to inhibit reticuloendothelial function, temporarily allowing prolonged platelet survival.

Immunosuppressive therapy. Treatment with many immunosuppressive agents (azathioprine, cyclophosphamide, vincristine, vinblastine) elicits occasional responses in refractory patients.

Mild ITP. There exists a group of patients with mild chronic immune thrombocytopenia (platelet counts 40–120,000) who do not bleed and who do not progress to develop another disease process. The natural history seems benign and patient reassurance should be the treatment.

"Wet ITP." Some patients with immune thrombocytopenia appear to have more vigorous bleeding at a given platelet count than the usual patient. In some patients, the antibody may affect platelet function as well as cause thrombocytopenia. Many hematologists treat patients who demonstrate impressive skin and mucous membrane bleeding more vigorously than the usual patient. There are little hard data, however, that such patients are more likely to have life-threatening bleeding.

Heparin Thrombocytopenia. Approximately 5% of patients receiving heparin develop thrombocytopenia. Most develop it while receiving therapeutic doses of heparin, but thrombocytopenia can be seen in patients with prophylactic doses following catheter flushes with as little as 100 units of heparin and even with heparin-impregnated catheters. Two separate syndromes are seen, although initially knowing which one is present is difficult.

1. **Mild thrombocytopenia** occurring early after starting heparin. Counts may drop daily, but remain above 50,000. Counts may normalize even when heparin is continued. Not associated with thrombosis. May not be immune in etiology. Mild thrombocytopenia occurs in approximately 5% of patients who receive heparin. Heparin may be cautiously continued with close monitoring of the platelet count.

2. **More severe and precipitous thrombocytopenia** usually occurs a few days later in the course of heparin, frequently dropping to less than 50,000/μl. It is sometimes associated

with the life-threatening syndrome of **heparin thrombosis** (seen in only a small fraction of those patients developing thrombocytopenia on heparin). Probably being seen less since Coumadin is now started earlier along with heparin, leading to shorter courses of heparin. Heparin should be stopped immediately if count drops to less than 50,000/μl. IV gamma globulin and plasmapheresis may be helpful for thrombocytopenic bleeding.

HIV-Associated Thrombocytopenia. Thrombocytopenia is a common presenting feature of HIV infection and develops with time in a significant number of HIV-positive persons before the occurrence of AIDS. It is frequently mild, and may spontaneously remit without treatment. The mechanism is a combination of immune destruction and decrease in production of platelets (normal or increased megakaryocytes on bone marrow exam). Often no treatment is required, except in hemophiliacs where platelet counts should probably be kept greater than 50,000/μl. Treatment with zidovudine is usually successful in increasing platelet production. When necessary, steroids are effective but usually require maintenance, which increases the infection risk. Splenectomy is frequently successful and seems to be safe.

Decreased Platelet Production (Table 8.6)

Routine Database

- The platelet count may be mildly or severely depressed.
- The peripheral smear usually reveals small isolated platelets.

Table 8.6
Production Thrombocytopenia: Differential Diagnosis

Myelophthisis (marrow replacement: tumor, fibrosis)
Primary bone marrow disorders (leukemia, myelodysplasia, myeloma, lymphoma)
Infection
Drugs

Platelets may be large and appear morphologically bizarre in some of the leukemias and the myelodysplastic syndromes.

- The bone marrow reveals decreased or absent megakaryocytes and may be diagnostic of a specific etiology (e.g., aplastic anemia, myelodysplasia, acute leukemia).

1. Myelophthisis.   Solid tumors metastatic to the bone marrow usually do not result in thrombocytopenia. However, when marrow metastases are extensive, as in breast, prostate, or metastatic oat cell cancer, platelet counts may fall late in the course of the illness. Some infiltrative marrow diseases (e.g., Gaucher's disease) result in thrombocytopenia because of hypersplenism rather than decreased platelet production. Thrombocytopenia resulting from myelophthisis is usually seen only with extensive marrow involvement, and leukoerythroblastosis is common on smear (p. 63). Thrombocytopenia is usually not severe enough to require platelet transfusion, and treatment is directed toward the underlying disorder.

2. Primary Bone Marrow Disorders.   Chronic myeloproliferative diseases such as polycythemia vera, primary thrombocythemia, and chronic granulocytic leukemia usually cause thrombocytosis, not thrombocytopenia. Patients with primary myelofibrosis may have normal platelet numbers, thrombocytopenia, or thrombocytosis. Acute leukemias, chronic lymphocytic leukemia, multiple myeloma, and leukemic reticuloendotheliosis may all be associated with a production megakaryocytic thrombocytopenia. Aplastic anemia is associated with severe production thrombocytopenia.

Treatment.   It is this category of production thrombocytopenias in which severe thrombocytopenia with bleeding may occur. The treatment is platelet transfusion. In the past routine prophylactic transfusion at a given platelet count (e.g., $<20,000/\mu l$) was practiced, but, depending on the clinical setting, transfusions are more appropriately administered based on clinical bleeding rather than a given count. In the bleeding patient, platelets may need to be transfused daily. Platelet increments following transfusion are decreased in the setting of bleeding, fever, infection, or sensitization. A number of platelet products can be used (p. 139).

3. Infection.   Infections, especially viral infections, routinely result in decreased platelet production. Mild thrombocytopenias are common, especially in children, with many viral illnesses. Occasionally thrombocytopenia is due to peripheral destruction from antibody as well. Bacterial infections may also result in decreased platelet production as well as increased sequestration with sepsis.

4. Drugs.   Alcohol is perhaps the most common drug cause of production thrombocytopenia. High alcohol intake may cause a severe thrombocytopenia. There is a return to normal within 7 to 10 days of discontinuation. Other mechanisms of thrombocytopenia in the alcoholic include folic acid deficiency and hypersplenism secondary to liver disease. Thiazides may rarely be associated with an antibody-mediated destructive thrombocytopenia. More commonly one sees a mild production thrombocytopenia, which usually returns to normal rapidly once the drug is discontinued. Other agents have occasionally been implicated as the etiology of isolated production thrombocytopenia.

Other drug-induced production thrombocytopenias are usually associated with leukopenia and anemia as well: cancer chemotherapeutic agents; immunosuppressive agents; gold; and the rare idiosyncratic reactions leading to aplastic anemia.

Ineffective Platelet Production

In conditions associated with ineffective megakaryocytopoiesis, megakaryocytes are present in the bone marrow, but platelet production is defective. The most common examples are megaloblastic anemia due to folate or B_{12} deficiency and drug-induced megaloblastosis. In these disorders there is classically a pancytopenia with a hypercellular, but qualitatively abnormal, bone marrow. Defective cell production leads to intramarrow destruction of precursor cells and defective delivery of platelets, white cells, and red cells to the periphery.

Hazards of Invasive Procedures in Patients with Thrombocytopenia

It is difficult to make generalizations about the relative hazards of biopsies and other invasive procedures in patients who are thrombocytopenic; the following are offered as guidelines only:

1. Open biopsies are generally safer than needle biopsies because of the ability to visually inspect for bleeding.
2. In the absence of a concomitant clotting problem or a problem with platelet function, a platelet count greater than 50,000 is usually associated with adequate platelet hemostatic plug function.
3. Even with higher platelet counts, be watchful if the patient demonstrates evidence of bleeding from venipunctures, etc., or has a concomitant clotting problem (e.g., DIC or liver disease).
4. Platelet counts less than 50,000/μl. Bleeding from procedures is more likely to occur in patients with production thrombocytopenias (leukemia, aplasia, myelophthisis) than thrombocytopenia due to increased platelet destruction or sequestration (e.g., ITP or hypersplenism).
5. Lumbar puncture and needle organ biopsies (lung, liver, kidneys, etc.) are more hazardous than thoracentesis, paracentesis, bone marrow aspirate, and biopsy; "need to know" must be carefully assessed in terms of risk/benefit considerations. In production thrombocytopenia and platelet counts less than 50,000/μl, platelet transfusions are indicated prior to, and possibly for several days following LP and organ biopsies.
6. Diagnostic needle biopsy procedures are hazardous in patients with platelet dysfunction, no matter what the platelet count (p. 101).

Summary

Remember:

1. In severe thrombocytopenia (< 10,000–20,000/ul) think of:
   a. Immune thrombocytopenia.
   b. Aplastic anemia.
   c. Acute leukemia and other causes of severe bone marrow replacement.

2. Large and frequently elongated platelets seen on a finger stick smear are usually young platelets, and their presence suggests a destructive/sequestration mechanism for the thrombocytopenia.

3. The degree of bleeding at any given platelet count varies with mechanism.

   a. Production thrombocytopenia will frequently demon-strate significant bleeding with counts less than 30,000, whereas destructive/sequestration thrombocytopenias may not bleed at much lower counts. This feature is nicely demonstrated by the relationship of bleeding time (p. 102) and platelet count in the two mechanisms. The aplastic anemia patient with 10,000 platelets will have a markedly prolonged bleeding time, whereas the ITP pa-tient with 10,000 platelets may have a normal bleeding time. The explanation for this variability is thought to be related to the functional superiority of young platelets compared to old platelets. In any event, the clinician is much more concerned about the likelihood of signifi-cant bleeding in severe production thrombocytopenia than in severe destruction/sequestration thrombocy-topenia.

4. Platelet transfusions are used for severe production throm-bocytopenia. They are not helpful, as a rule, in destruc-tion/sequestration thrombocytopenia.

5. Fibrinolytic inhibitors (epsilon amino caproic acid) can sometimes be helpful in bleeding, thrombocytopenic pa-tients refractory to platelet transfusions.

6. We have more platelets than needed. Hemostasis approaches normal at platelet counts greater than 50,000 in production thrombocytopenia and at lower counts in destruction/se-questration thrombocytopenia.

DISORDERS OF PLATELET FUNCTION

Hemostatic-plug type clinical bleeding in the absence of throm-bocytopenia raises the suspicion of the presence of an abnor-mality of platelet function. The further database for a suspected disorder of platelet function frequently begins with a bleeding time.

Bleeding Time

The bleeding time is a gross in vivo test of hemostatic plug function. Bleeding times based on the template method are accurate, and disposable devices are commercially available. There is poor correlation between the degree of prolongation of the bleeding time and the degree of clinical bleeding, but the test is useful as a means of diagnosing platelet dysfunction.

The test is relatively insensitive to platelet dysfunction as many patients with congenital and acquired platelet dysfunction will have normal bleeding times. However, most patients who have spontaneous bleeding or a major bleeding risk with surgery will have a prolonged bleeding time. The bleeding time, however, is not a reliable indication of the degree of risk of bleeding with surgery. Many patients with platelet dysfunction and a prolonged bleeding time do not bleed with surgery, and the likelihood of bleeding does not correlate with the degree of prolongation of the bleeding time. Patient history is more useful in this regard. The bleeding time is not recommended as a screening test before surgery or invasive diagnostic procedures.

Normal Platelet Function

After vascular injury, platelets adhere to subendothelial tissue through the bridging action of von Willebrand factor (produced in endothelial cells and megakaryocytes) between tissue and platelet membrane glycoproteins. Arachidonic acid is released from platelet phospholipids leading to the generation of thromboxane A_2 in the platelet (inhibited by aspirin in small doses), and prostacyclin generation in the endothelium (inhibited by aspirin in larger doses). Subsequently, there is stimulation of the release reaction of platelet-dense body constituents (most notably ADP) resulting in the continued aggregation of more platelets at the site, and the release of α granule contents (fibrinogen, vWF, platelet factor 4, etc.). Further recruitment of platelets follows with a conformational change in platelet membrane glycoprotein

Iib/IIIa. This leads to exposure of a receptor for fibrinogen and a catalytic surface for the coagulation cascade. Thrombin generation leads to further platelet aggregation and localizing clotting.

Disorders of Platelet Function

Congenital causes of abnormal platelet function are rare (except for von Willebrand's disease). Some of the syndromes include:

  a. **von Willebrand's disease** (p. 121).
  b. **Bernard-Soulier syndrome:** An autosomal recessive disease characterized by large, bizarre platelet morphology, mild thrombocytopenia, and defective platelet adhesion secondary to membrane glycoprotein Ib/IX abnormalities.
  c. **Glanzmann's thrombasthenia:** Autosomal recessive disease associated with absent clot retraction and abnormal platelet aggregation due to membrane glycoprotein IIb/IIIa abnormalities.
  d. **Disorders of platelet release reaction:** A heterogeneous group of disorders characterized by defective platelet aggregation.

Acquired disorders of platelet function are much more common: (Table 8.7)

  a. **Drugs:** Many drugs alter platelet function in vitro, but only

Table 8.7
Acquired Causes of Bleeding Secondary to Platelet Dysfunction

Chronic myeloproliferative disease
Acute leukemia
Myelodysplastic syndromes
Uremia
Liver disease
Antibodies to platelets (e.g., ITP)
Dysproteinemia
DIC
Cardiopulmonary bypass
Blood bank storage defect
Acquired von Willebrand's disease
Acquired storage pool disease
Drugs (principally ASA & Ticlopidine)

aspirin [acetylsalicylic acid (ASA)] and ticlopidine hydrochloride consistently prolong the bleeding time and cause clinical bleeding. ASA interferes with platelet function by inhibiting prostaglandin synthesis and the formation of thromboxane A_2. An increase in bleeding time is seen in normal people following the ingestion of aspirin. Aspirin also accentuates the bleeding time prolongation in many patients with underlying disorders of platelet function and should not be given to patients with known bleeding disorders. Ticlopidine, approved in the US for stroke prevention in patients intolerant to ASA, interferes with platelet aggregation. Its effect is additive with ASA. High doses of some beta lactam antibiotics may cause clinical bleeding associated with a prolonged bleeding time, especially in patients with renal failure or mild thrombocytopenia. Alcohol may cause prolongation of the bleeding time. Other drugs reported to occasionally prolong the bleeding time include indomethacin, naproxen, ε-aminocaproic acid (large doses), mithramycin, nitrofurantoin, halothane and prostacyclin. Although non-steroidal, anti-inflammatory drugs interfere with platelet function in vitro, except for aspirin, they usually do not cause clinical bleeding.

b. **Uremia:** Bleeding time prolongation associated with platelet dysfunction is seen in severe uremia (dialysis patients). Multiple possible mechanisms have been identified. Dialysis (peritoneal or hemodialysis) is the treatment of choice for severe hemostatic plug-type bleeding in patients with renal failure. Of interest is the direct effect of the hematocrit on the bleeding time in uremia (and normals). It is felt that the incidence of severe uremic bleeding has decreased since the institution of erythropoietin therapy. An HCT of 30% is sufficient to improve the bleeding time. Short-term correction of the bleeding time and decreased clinical bleeding may be achieved by the administration of 1-deamino-8-D-arginine vasopressin (**DDAVP**), which causes the release of large molecular weight vWF from endothelial cells. Subcutaneous or intravenous administration results in a rapid effect which lasts only a few hours. Continued administration beyond 2–3 days usually is ineffective owing to tachyphylaxis. Rare arterial thrombosis following DDAVP has been reported and caution, especially in the elderly, should be exercised. There are reports of the usefulness of **conjugated estrogen** in correcting uremic bleeding and long bleeding times. Intravenous administration may result in an effect in a few days and may last for up to 2 weeks. **Cryoprecipitate** (perhaps as a source of vWF) may also be helpful.

c. **Cardiopulmonary bypass surgery:** A significant bleeding time prolongation occurs during cardiopulmonary bypass. Only a small fraction of patients demonstrate increased postoperative bleeding. When clinical bleeding occurs, platelet transfusion and DDAVP are useful.

d. **Miscellaneous:** Platelet dysfunction is seen in some patients with severe liver disease (perhaps related to high levels of fibrinogen/fibrin degradation products), patients with multiple myeloma and other dysproteinemias (proteins interfering with platelet function), and in some patients with leukemia (abnormal platelet function). Patients with chronic myeloproliferative disorders and elevated platelet counts also have functionally abnormal platelets.

THROMBOCYTOSIS

Table 8.8 lists the common etiologies of thrombocytosis. Chronic myeloproliferative disorders may be associated with platelet counts greater than 1,000,000 per μl. The platelets are morphologically bizarre and functionally abnormal. Abnormal morphology is more common in polycythemia vera, primary myelofibrosis, and primary thrombocythemia than in chronic granulocytic leukemia. Bleeding is common in such patients, usually when the platelet count is high. The platelets also tend to clump in the microcirculation and may contribute to the thrombotic problems seen in these patients. Many recommend treatment to decrease the platelet count in such patients (hydroxyurea), although proof of efficacy is difficult to determine. Secondary thrombocytosis does not cause a bleeding diathesis or thrombosis.

Table 8.8
Thrombocytosis: Differential Diagnosis

Myeloproliferative Disorders (frequently >1,000,000)

 Polycythemia vera
 Primary thrombocythemia
 Agnogenic myeloid metaplasia
 Chronic granulocytic leukemia

Secondary Thrombocytosis

 Inflammation
 Malignancy
 Hodgkin's disease
 Acute bleeding
 Postsplenectomy
 Rebound from severe thrombocytopenia
 Severe iron deficiency

Nonthrombocytopenic Purpura with Normal Platelet Function

Many of the following disorders are associated with skin and/or mucous membrane hemorrhage suggestive of a hemostatic plug-type bleeding defect. However, others are associated with ecchymoses and confluent lesions more suggestive of a coagulation problem.

Senile purpura

Steroid purpura

Connective tissue disorders (Ehlers-Danlos syndrome, pseudoxanthoma elasticum)

Scurvy

Amyloidosis

Dysproteinemias

Allergic purpura

Autoerythrocyte sensitization.

Suggested Reading

Bell WR, Braine HG, Ness PM, Kickler TS. Improved survival in thrombotic thrombocytopenic purpura-hemolytic uremic syndrome: clinical experience in 108 patients. N Engl J Med 1991;325:398–403.

Cohen I, Gardner FH. Thrombocytopenia as a laboratory sign and complication of gram negative bacteremia infection. Arch Intern Med 1966; 117:112.

Cowan DH, Henes JD. Thrombocytopenia of severe alcoholism. Ann Intern Med 1971;74:37.

Dawson RB, Brown JA, Mahalati K, et. al. Durable remissions following prolonged plasma exchange in thrombotic thrombocytopenic purpura. Journal of Clinical Apheresis 1994:9:112–115.

George JN, El-Harake MA, Aster RH. Thrombocytopenia due to enhanced platelet destruction by immunologic mechanisms. In: Beutler E, Lichtman MA, Coller BS, Kipps TJ, eds. Williams Hematology. New York: McGraw-Hill, 1995:1315–1355.

George JN, El-Harake MA. Thrombocytopenia due to enhanced platelet destruction by nonimmunologic mechanisms. In: Beutler E, Lichtman MA, Coller BS, Kipps TJ, eds. Williams Hematology. New York: McGraw-Hill, 1995;1290–1315.

George JN, Shattil SJ. The clinical importance of acquired abnormalities of platelet function. N Engl J Med 1991;324:27.

Lind SE. The bleeding time does not predict surgical bleeding. Blood 1991;77:2547–2552.

Warkentiin TE, Kelton JG. Heparin and platelets. Hematology/Oncology Clinics of North America 1990;4:243–264.

Chapter 9

Disorders Of Clotting

Based on the results of the initial database discussed in Chapter 7, the diagnostic focus narrows. This chapter deals with disorders of clotting, without evidence of an associated platelet problem.

ISOLATED PROLONGATION OF THE PARTIAL THROMBIN TIME (PTT) [NORMAL PROTHROMBIN TIME (PT), THROMBIN TIME (TT) AND PLATELET COUNT, FIG. 9.1]
Differential Diagnosis

- Spurious
- Circulating anticoagulant
- von Willebrand's disease
- Hemophilia A and B
- Congenital deficiency of Factors XI and XII
- Congenital deficiency of high-molecular-weight kininogen and prekallikrein
- Constant infusion heparin

Spurious

An unexpected prolongation of the PTT is usually **spurious** and the test should be repeated with attention to proper filling of the citrate tube; the ratio of anticoagulant to blood is important as is rapid transport to the lab for assay. If the PTT is still abnormal, it must be explained even in the absence of a history of bleeding (see hemophilia below).

Circulating Anticoagulant

Differential Diagnosis

- Hemophilia A and B
- Postpartum
- Elderly
- SLE and other autoimmune diseases
- Drugs (chlorpromazine, penicillin)
- No apparent reason

Acquired inhibitors of coagulation factors may develop in the hemophiliac who has received multiple transfusions (anti VIII/anti IX), and result in severe bleeding refractory to factor replacement. Treatment usually requires use of concentrates containing activated Factor X. Inhibitors may develop spontaneously in patients with lupus or other collagen vascular diseases, in women during pregnancy or postpartum, rarely during the administration of various drugs, and occasionally, in the el-

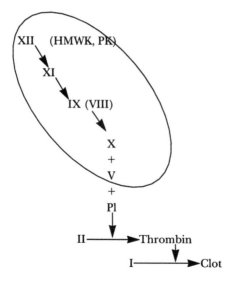

Figure 9.1. Partial thromboplastin time.

derly. These inhibitors are usually directed against Factor VIII, but occasionally against Factor IX, XI or V. Acquired anti Factor VIII inhibitors may be associated with massive spontaneous hemorrhage and treatment is difficult (Factor VIII replacement for low titer inhibitors and activated Factor X concentrates or porcine Factor VIII for high titer inhibitors). Unlike inhibitors developing in hemophiliacs, immunosuppressant therapy may be successful in controlling spontaneously developing inhibitors.

The **lupus anticoagulant** is an acquired inhibitor directed against phospholipids (p. 125). When routine coagulation tests are affected by the lupus anticoagulant, the most typical pattern is a significant prolongation of the PTT and little or no prolongation of the PT. The inhibitor is seen in patients with lupus and testing frequently reveals a biologic false-positive test for syphilis, thrombocytopenia, and anticardiolipin antibodies. The inhibitor is also found in other clinical settings [autoimmune diseases, drugs (phenothiazines), and in patients with no apparent disease]. Patients with the lupus anticoagulant do not have a bleeding diathesis but rather a tendency to thrombosis.

Diagnosis:

- Mixing studies of patient and normal plasma to see if patient plasma prolongs the PTT of normal plasma
- **Factor Assay** when inhibitor is associated with bleeding (most are anti Factor VIII antibodies)
- Titer of the inhibitor
- When a lupus anticoagulant is expected, other tests are needed, e.g., **Russell's viper venom time** (p. 125), for confirmation

von Willebrand's Disease

Von Willebrand's disease (p. 121) classically results in a prolonged bleeding time as well as in decreased Factor VIII activity (prolonged PTT). Diagnosis is usually helped by a family history suggesting an autosomal dominant inheritance pattern and by a bleeding pattern suggesting a "hemostatic plug" formation defect in contrast to the bleeding pattern of the hemophiliac.

Hemophilia and Other Congenital Abnormalities of Coagulation

Approximately 85% of patients have Factor VIII deficiency, 12% have decreased Factor IX activity, and 1% have Factor XI deficiency. Deficiencies of Factor XII, High-molecular-weight kininogen and prekallikrein deficiency are very rare and not associated with bleeding. About 50% of patients with Factor VIII deficiency are severe (< 2% activity) and are diagnosed in infancy. However, mild cases (5–20% activity) may be seen in persons who reach adulthood without serious bleeding. Such patients may have life-threatening bleeding with trauma or surgery; hence, the obvious importance of explaining an unexpected prolongation of the PTT. The PTT is sensitive enough to detect procoagulant levels below 25% activity.

Modern concentrates of Factors VIII and IX are practically free of viral contamination and recombinant Factor VIII is now available. Factor VIII concentrates have essentially replaced cryoprecipitate in the treatment of Factor VIII deficiency.

Constant Infusion Heparin

Additional Database

An unexpected prolongation of the PTT might reasonably initiate the following workup:

    a. Repeat to rule out a spurious prolongation of the PTT
    b. Screen for a circulating anticoagulant (inhibitor)
    c. If b. is positive and there is no clinical bleeding, test for the presence of the lupus anticoagulant.
    d. If b. is positive and there is clinical bleeding, use Factor VIII assay and titer of the inhibitor.
    e. If b. is negative, test to differentiate von Willebrand's disease from hemophilia (p.121).

ISOLATED PROLONGATION OF THE PT OR PT PLUS PTT (NORMAL TT AND PLATELET COUNT, FIG. 9.2)
Differential Diagnosis

- Coumarin anticoagulation
- Vitamin K deficiency
- Drugs

- Liver disease
- Rare congenital coagulation defects
- Circulating anticoagulant (SLE)
- Chronic DIC
- Excessive heparinization
- Aspirin

Coumadin Anticoagulation and Vitamin K Deficiency (p. 134)

Drugs

A number of drugs may cause hypoprothrombinemia manifested by a prolongation of the PT or the PT and PTT. The most common association has been with the β-lactam antibiotics. Those reported to occasionally cause significant bleeding diathesis include cefamandole and cefoperazone. A large number of other drugs augment the effect of warfarin by altering its metabolism. Many antibiotics may precipitate vitamin K deficiency by altering gut flora and in vivo production of vitamin K.

Liver Disease

Early hepatocellular disease may cause prolongation of the PT mainly due to a decrease in Factor VII production. With further worsening of liver function, the PTT may become abnormal as well. Only in endstage liver disease do fibrinogen levels fall sig-

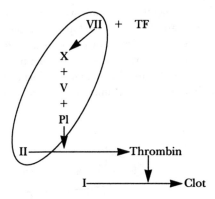

Figure 9.2. Prothrombin time.

nificantly. In very severe hepatocellular disease the TT may be prolonged because of the liver's inability to clear fibrin split products, and a picture which suggests DIC may be seen (p. 117).

Congenital Coagulation Defects

Congenital deficiencies of Factor VII, Factor X, Factor V and Factor II occur rarely.

Circulating Anticoagulant

The lupus anticoagulant described above usually causes an isolated prolongation of the PTT, but sometimes causes a prolongation of both PTT and PT. Circulating anticoagulants directed against Factor V also cause prolongation of both tests.

DIC (p. 117)

Heparin (p. 132)

Aspirin

Salicylates in large doses may prolong the PT, and sometimes the PTT, probably because of an effect on prothrombin synthesis. Vitamin K prevents the abnormality. Bleeding is uncommon.

PROLONGED PT, PTT AND TT
(NORMAL PLATELETS, FIG. 9.3)

Third-stage coagulation problems characteristically prolong the TT. The PT and PTT are also abnormal because the endpoint of all three tests requires a normal third stage for clot formation. Depending on the method, the thrombin time may be less sensitive than the PT and PTT and may be normal in some situations where there is abnormal third-stage coagulation.

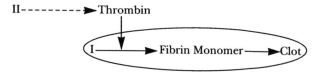

Figure 9.3.   Thrombin time.

Differential Diagnosis

- Afibrinogenemia (hypofibrinogenemia)
- Dysfibrinogenemia
- High-dose heparin
- DIC
- Fibrinolysis
- Severe liver disease
- Dysproteinemia

Afibrinogenemia and Hypofibrinogenemia

These are rare hereditary disorders of blood coagulation. Severe hypofibrinogenemia may also be acquired secondary to fulminant acute intravascular clotting as in obstetric emergencies (retained dead fetus, amniotic fluid embolism).

Dysfibrinogenemia

Functionally abnormal fibrinogens occur as uncommon congenital disorders and may occasionally be seen as acquired problems in liver disease (especially hepatomas).

High Dose Heparin (p. 132)

DIC (p. 117)

Fibrinolysis (p. 118)

Severe Liver Disease (p. 113)

Dysproteinemia

Some patients with large concentrations of monoclonal proteins (myeloma, macroglobulinemia) develop coagulopathies secondary to inhibition by the protein of various steps in coagulation. Third-stage inhibition is most common, although any pattern, as well as platelet dysfunction, can be seen.

Hazards of Invasive Procedures

In general, invasive diagnostic or therapeutic procedures carry a significant risk of bleeding in patients with any of the above clotting disorders. Abnormalities of the PT, PTT, or TT should be respected. A specific diagnosis should be pursued, appropriate consultation obtained, and indicated therapy instituted prior to invasive procedures.

Suggested Reading

Hoyer LW. Acquired anticoagulants. In: Beutler E, Lichtman MA, Coller BS, Kipps TJ, eds. Williams Hematology. New York: McGraw-Hill, 1995:1485–1496.

Roberts HR, Hoffman M. Hemophilia and related conditions—inherited deficiencies of prothrombin (Factor II), Factor V, and Factors VII to XII. In: Beutler E, Lichtman MA, Coller BS, Kipps TJ, eds. Williams Hematology. New York: McGraw-Hill, 1995:1413–1439.

Suchman AC, Griner PF. Diagnostic uses of the activated partial thromboplastin time and prothrombin time. Ann Intern Med 1986;104: 810

Chapter 10

Conditions Associated with Abnormalities of Both Clotting and Platelets

During the workup of a patient for bleeding diathesis, finding evidence of abnormalities involving both clotting and platelets (quantitative or qualitative) suggests the presence of one of the following clinical problems:

DIFFERENTIAL DIAGNOSIS

- Disseminated intravascular coagulation (DIC)
- Alcohol
- Liver disease
- von Willebrand's disease
- Dilution coagulopathy

DISSEMINATED INTRAVASCULAR COAGULATION

Intravascular clotting may be initiated by release of thromboplastic substances into the circulation, activating clotting as, for example, in malignancy or tissue ischemia secondary to hypotension. Platelets are usually consumed in the clotting process. DIC may occur as an acute event or as a more chronic ongoing phenomenon.

ACUTE DIC

Acute DIC is usually severe, with possible significant clinical bleeding.

Laboratory Features

a. Various clotting factors are consumed (I, V, VIII, XIII)
b. Platelets are consumed, and thrombocytopenia may be severe.
c. Secondary fibrinolysis occurs.

Circulating plasminogen is activated to the enzyme plasmin, which digests fibrinogen and fibrin (as well as other coagulation factors, e.g., V and VIII), resulting in:

Fibrinogen degradation products (FDPs)
Fibrin degradation products (fdps)
D-dimer products

FDPs/fdps circulate until cleared by the liver. They may be measured in vitro by one of several techniques. The products themselves interfere with normal clot formation by acting as antithrombins and interfering with normal fibrin polymerization. They may also interfere with normal platelet function. The **D-dimer** products result from the degredation of cross-linked fibrin and is a sensitive test for DIC (secondary fibrinolysis). However it may be positive in other settings of intravascular clot formation (e.g., venous thrombosis) in the absence of DIC.

Table 10.1
Differential Diagnosis of Acute DIC

Obstetrics
  Retained dead fetus
  Amniotic fluid embolism
  Abruptio placentae
  Fatty liver of pregnancy
  Induced abortion

Infection (bacterial, viral, rickettsial, mycotic, protozoal)
Shock
Acute progranulocytic leukemia
Hemolytic transfusion reactions
Heat stroke
Tissue necrosis

The bleeding in acute DIC results from a combination of problems:

1. Clotting factor consumption
2. Thrombocytopenia
3. Production of FDPs/fdps that act as anticoagulants

Common Laboratory Database

1. Prothrombin time (PT)—abnormal
2. Partial thromboplastin time (PTT)—abnormal
3. Thrombin time (TT)—abnormal
4. Thrombocytopenia
5. Elevated levels of FDPs/fdps
6. Elevated D-dimer
7. RBC fragmentation (from fibrin deposition in arterioles) occurs in a minority of cases

Once the process of intravascular clotting is stopped (usually by eliminating the underlying cause), a rapid reversal of the abnormal laboratory tests occurs. The PT, PTT and TT may return to normal in a matter of hours, and FDPs/fdps are rapidly cleared by the liver. The platelet count returns to normal more slowly (over several days).

SUBACUTE DIC

Less fulminant intravascular clotting may occur in all of the causes of DIC listed above. In such cases the abnormalities seen in the laboratory data are quite variable, and the diagnosis becomes more difficult. Most hematologists require at least the following laboratory abnormalities for diagnosis:

1. Decrease in the fibrinogen concentration
2. Mild thrombocytopenia
3. Elevated FDPs/fdps
4. Increased D-dimer

CHRONIC DIC

The best clinical example of chronic DIC is metastatic cancer. Low levels of ongoing intravascular clotting probably explain other hypercoagulable phenomena seen frequently in cancer patients, namely, migrating thrombophlebitis and marantic endocarditis. The process of DIC in such patients may be mild and compensated, and clinical bleeding is infrequent. Diagnosis may be difficult.

Routine Laboratory Tests

1. PT—normal or slightly abnormal
2. PTT—normal or slightly abnormal
3. TT—normal or slightly abnormal
4. Platelet count—frequently normal or even elevated
5. FDPs/fdps—elevated
6. D-dimer—elevated

Remember that less fulminant DIC may be hard to diagnose and may result in only minor routine laboratory abnormalities. Extremely low-grade DIC may only be detected by sensitive tests of fibrinogen and platelet survival. Less fulminant DIC may be extremely difficult to distinguish from liver disease or from the dilution coagulopathy seen in the massively transfused patient.

TREATMENT

By far the most important treatment is that directed at the cause. Treat the shock, sepsis, evacuate the dead fetus, etc. Intravascular coagulation may be interrupted by heparin administration, which acts as an antithrombin and inhibits Factor X activation. Once clot formation is stopped, fibrinolysis ceases and FDPs/fdps are no longer formed. Replacement therapy in patients with severe thrombocytopenia and hypofibrinogenemia is usually recommended with significant bleeding or if surgery is needed. Platelets and fresh frozen plasma, or cryoprecipitate if the hypofibrinogenemia is severe, are given. Heparin is usually recommended in patients with thrombotic complications of DIC (e.g., digital ischemia in purpura fulminans, thromboembolism). Its use in other causes of DIC is controversial. As noted, the diagnosis is difficult in subacute or chronic cases. Acute cases are rapidly reversible by treatment of the underlying cause.

LIVER DISEASE AND ALCOHOL

Abnormalities of both clotting and platelets are common in acute liver disease and/or alcoholism. Bleeding may occur for several reasons:

1. Decreased production of factors made in the liver (II, VII, V, IX, X).
2. Decreased production of vitamin K factors in obstructive jaundice (II, VII, IX, X).
3. Low-grade DIC with decreased clearance of FDPs/fdps.
4. Thrombocytopenia from:
    a. Hypersplenism
    b. DIC
    c. ETOH alone
    d. Folate deficiency, especially in the alcoholic.

VON WILLEBRAND'S DISEASE

This is an autosomal-dominant disease with significant variability in degree of clinical bleeding. The bleeding pattern is more like that of a hemostatic plug defect than a clotting problem, with gastrointestinal bleeding being most common. Hemarthroses are not seen.

Pathophysiology

Functional Factor VIII results from the interaction of two molecular complexes, one x-linked defective in Hemophilia A and one under autosomal control (Factor VIII/von Willebrand Factor, F VIII/vWF) which is abnormal in von Willebrand's disease. F VIII/vWF is produced by the endothelial lining cells of blood vessels and is necessary for normal platelet/endothelial cell interaction. Von Willebrand's disease is not a single entity. Quantitative (Type I) and Qualitative (Types II A and B) abnormalities in F VIII/vWF have been described, as well as a number of other variants.

Routine Laboratory Findings

- Prolonged bleeding time. Accentuated by aspirin.
- Frequently, although not always, prolonged PTT.
- Normal PT, TT, platelet count.

Specialized Laboratory Tests

- Plasma Factor VIII procoagulant (VIII.C) activity (decreased in Type I disease; normal or decreased in Type II A and II B disease).
- Plasma Factor VIII antigen (VIII:Ag) activity (decreased in Type I; normal or decreased in Types IIA and IIB).
- von Willebrand factor antigen (vWF:Ag)
- Ristocetin cofactor activity (decreased in Types I and II A and usually decreased in Type II B).
- Electrophoresis of F VIII/vWF by various techniques.

Treatment

Fresh frozen plasma (FFP) and cryoprecipitate are frequently effective in correcting the PTT and bleeding time abnormalities and the clinical bleeding. Most Factor VIII **concentrates** do not correct the platelet function abnormality, but there now exist several concentrates that contain therapeutic amounts of vWF. Cryoprecipitate as the treatment of choice for severe bleeding in patients with von Willebrand's disease has been replaced by concentrates. **Cryoprecipitate** remains a useful treatment for moderate to severe bleeding. The amount necessary varies from patient to patient. Commonly 6 to 12 units given daily or every other day are required. Infusion of 1-deamino-8-D-arginine vasopressin (**DDAVP**) increases the plasma concentration of F VIII/vWF and may temporarily correct the bleeding diathesis in some patients (especially Type I) with von Willebrand's disease. ϵ-aminocaproic acid (ϵ-ACA), an inhibitor of fibrinolysis, may be useful in preventing bleeding from minor surgery and tooth extractions.

DILUTION COAGULOPATHY

This problem is seen particularly in trauma patients undergoing massive transfusions with banked blood. Blood refrigerated in the blood bank for 10 days to 3 weeks becomes depleted of:

- Functioning platelets (depleted in 1 day)
- Factor VIII
- Factor V

Dilution in vivo of platelets and Factors V and VIII may result in:

- Thrombocytopenia
- Prolongation of PT
- Prolongation of PTT
- Associated clinical bleeding

Comments

Actually, in the controlled setting of hypertransfusion (e.g., open heart surgery), it is unusual to see marked thrombocytopenia, a significant prolongation of the PT and PTT, and clinical bleeding, even with massive transfusion. In the trauma patient in shock, one sees more abnormal numbers and a more significant bleeding diathesis, usually because DIC is also present and diagnostically difficult to distinguish from dilution coagulopathy. Fresh frozen plasma (a source of Factors V and VIII) and platelets are best administered in these settings only when significantly abnormal tests are encountered rather than prophylactically (the latter being a common practice in massively transfused patients in years past).

Suggested Reading

Scott JP, Montgomery RR. Therapy of von Willebrand disease. Seminars in Thrombosis and Hemostasis 1993;19:37–47.

White GA, Montgomery RR. Clinical aspects of and therapy for von Willebrand disease. In: Hoffman R, Benz EJ, Shattil SJ, Furie B, Cohen HJ, Silberstein LE eds. Hematology: Basic Principles and Practice. New York: Churchill Livingstone, 1995:1725–1736.

Williams EC, Mosher DF. Disseminated intravascular coagulation. In: Hoffman R, Benz EF, Shattil SJ, Furie B, Cohen HJ, Silberstein LE eds. Hematology: Basic Principles and Practice. New York: Churchill Livingstone, 1995:1758–1769.

Chapter 11

Venous Thrombosis

PREDISPOSITION

Many predisposing events are known to increase the risk of venous thromboembolism, including stasis as with prolonged sitting, trauma, prolonged bedrest or inactivity, obesity, high dose estrogens, surgery, and congestive heart failure.

The occurrence of repeated episodes of thromboembolism or thrombosis without a known predisposing risk raises the question as to the presence of an underlying hypercoagulable state. Table 11.1 lists acquired causes of hypercoagulability and Table 11.2 lists congenital conditions associated with thrombosis.

There has been considerable development in the understanding of the mechanisms of the primary congenital causes of hypercoagulability, especially antithrombin III, Protein C, Protein S deficiency, and congenital resistance to activated Protein C.

Antiphospholipid Antibody Syndrome: Lupus Anticoagulants, Anticardiolipin Antibodies

Lupus anticoagulants (LA) are antibodies (usually IgG or IgM) which in vitro interfere with various coagulation tests which require phospholipid. Of the routine screening coagulation tests, classically the activated partial thromboplastin time (PTT) is prolonged, the prothrombin time (PT) is normal. Other coagulation tests also identify and confirm the presence of lupus anticoagulants. The most common are the dilute **Russell Viper Venom Time** (RVVT) and the **Kaolin clotting time** (KCT). These antibodies are identified as inhibitors in vitro by **mixing studies** in which normal plasma fails to correct the prolonged coagulation test.

Table 11.1
Acquired Causes of Hypercoagulability

Coagulation Abnormalities

Oral contraceptives
Pregnancy
Malignancy
Nephrotic syndrome
Lupus anticoagulants
Hyper homocysteinemia

Platelet Abnormalities

Myeloproliferative disorders
Paroxysmal nocturnal hemoglobinuria
Heparin thrombocytopenia
Diabetes mellitus

Abnormalities of Blood Vessels, Cells and Plasma

Stasis
Artificial valves, blood vessels
Thrombotic thrombocytopenic purpura
Hyperviscosity (SS disease, P Vera, monoclonal gammopathies,
leukemia with leukostasis)

In vivo, patients with LAs do not bleed, but many have a predisposition to arterial and/or venous thrombosis. Other antiphospholipid antibodies are seen in many of these patients and increased titre of anticardiolipin antibodies (ACAs) also identify possible predisposition to thrombosis.

Clinical Occurrence (LAs, ACAs)

Lupus	LAs in 30% of patients
Lupus	ACAs in 40% of patients
Lupus	Both (LA & ACA) in 35 to 90% of patients
Patients on Phenothiazines	LAs are common
Lymphoproliferative Disorders	increased incidence of LA
Other Autoimmune Disorders	increased incidence of LA
HIV	increased incidence of LA
Normals (especially elderly)	LAs in 1–2% of population

Table 11.2
Most Important Hereditary Causes of Hypercoagulability

Antithrombin III deficiency
Protein C deficiency
Protein S deficiency
Congenital resistance to activated Protein C

Incidence of Thrombotic Events

LAs in lupus	40%
ACAs in lupus	40%
Lupus without LA/ACA	15%
LAs in patients on phenothiazines	No increased risk
LAs/ACAS in patients without lupus	unclear, but less than in lupus
Patients with persistent LA/ACA and previous thrombotic event	50% chance of recurrence in 5 years
Lupus, LA/ACA +, pregnancy. Fetal loss secondary to placental thrombosis.	40% per pregnancy

Antithrombin III Deficiency

Antithrombin III deficiency is an autosomal dominant condition classically associated with a positive familial history, typically associated with deep venous thrombosis (DVT) (sometimes mesenteric vein thrombosis), occurring in early life, but not before puberty. About 50% of affected family members actually experience clinical thrombosis. There are two major types: **Type I**—Prevalence is 1 in 5000 and usually clinically significant due to quantitative decrease in functional inhibitor; **Type II**—Prevalence is 1 in 350 with most affected individuals not experiencing venous thrombosis. Multiple mutations affecting function have been identified and most seem not to be clinically important.

   Heparin cofactor assay is the most useful screen which will identify Type I- and Type II-affected individuals. **Immunologic assay of antigen** distinguishes between Type I and Type II defects and **progressive antithrombin assay** helps to separate Type II patients with clinically significant mutations from clinically insignificant ones.

Many conditions affect the level of antithrombin III. Diagnosis and treatment require consultation with a specialist in coagulation disorders.

Protein C Deficiency

Incidence may be as high as 1 in 200 persons. Usually autosomal dominant inheritance. The majority of patients with levels in the heterozygote range do not have an increased risk of thrombosis, so there are probably other unrecognized contributing factors in Protein C-deficient patients who develop thrombosis.

As with antithrombin III deficiency, quantitative deficiency **(Type I)** and functionally abnormal protein C **(Type II)** both occur. Type I deficiency is more common. Thrombotic problems may occur first at a young age (early 20s) or not be experienced until later in life. Thrombotic events are usually DVT or mesenteric vein thrombosis, but superficial thrombophlebitis is also common. Cerebral venous thrombosis and arterial stroke in young adults have also been reported.

Coumarin necrosis may occur in patients with protein C deficiency and known carriers should be heparinized before starting on low doses of coumarin. Approximately one-third of patients who develop coumarin necrosis are protein C deficient and reports of coumarin necrosis in affected individuals are uncommon. So protein C deficiency is not the complete story behind this rare complication of coumarin therapy.

Protein S Deficiency

Protein S deficiency is a necessary co-factor for the activity of Protein C and is clinically similar to Protein C and antithrombin III deficiencies.

Resistance to Activated Protein C

Resistance to activated Protein C is the most recently described and the most common of the congenital causes of hypercoagulability (perhaps 5% of population). Most cases are caused by a defect in Factor V which inhibits Protein C's inactivation of Factor V. Most persons with the defect do not have clinical problems.

Problems with Assays and Interpreting Test Results

The assays are difficult, require stringent quality control, need to be repeated, and are affected by a host of variables. The significance of abnormal test results in many patients and family members is unclear since many persons with low levels do not develop thrombosis. Interpretation of test results and further workup is best left to specialists with expertise in coagulation disorders.

It is important to follow strictly the procedural guides of the laboratory conducting the tests. In general it's best to draw assays before anticoagulation is started or after anticoagulation drugs are stopped. Antithrombin III should not be assayed in patients on heparin or with DIC, nephrosis, liver disease, or while on estrogens. Protein C and S optimally should not be drawn while patients are on coumadin, although some labs feel they can accurately correct results based on the degree of anticoagulation. Liver disease, DIC, estrogens, sepsis, ARDS, pregnancy, HIV, and other conditions may falsely affect one or both assays. The assay for Protein C resistance is difficult, not widely available, and must be conducted on patients without acute thrombosis and not taking anticoagulants. Research tests exist for the assay of Protein C resistance in patients on anticoagulants, but are not widely available.

Table 11.3
Congenital Hypercoagulable States

Candidates for Screening
Thrombosis occurring at a young age
Impressive family history
Thrombosis occurring at an unusual site
Recurrent thrombosis on anticoagulation
Warfarin-induced skin necrosis
Thrombosis occurring without obvious risk

Table 11.3 lists clinical settings where screening may be appropriate.

PREVENTION
Prevention In Moderate And High-Risk Settings

Moderate Risk: General surgery over age 40 or immobilization with severe medical illness.

1. Low dose heparin [5000 μl subcutaneously (sub q) every 8 to 12 hours], or intermittent pneumatic compression
2. For neurosurgery or GU surgery use intermittent pneumatic compression.

High Risk: Elective hip surgery, hip fracture, major knee surgery, or major general surgery.

1. Low molecular weight heparin or
2. Oral anticoagulants to International Normalization Ration (INR) of 2 or
3. Sub q heparin using dose to keep PTT at 1.2–1.5 times the baseline.

Low Molecular Weight Heparin (LMWH)

Currently (Spring 1996) in the US, LMWH is approved only for prophylaxis in patients undergoing hip replacement. However, LMWH is likely to replace standard heparin in increasing settings over the next few years. Recent data suggest that, in the treatment of thromboembolic disease, LMWH is at least as effective as standard heparin, is easier to give (sub q injection once or twice daily and with no need to monitor with coagulation tests), is associated with less clinical bleeding, and perhaps with less heparin-associated thrombocytopenia.

Heparin, Mechanism of Action
Standard Heparin

a. Inhibits equally Xa and thrombin
b. Thrombin inhibition requires large molecule which can bind to both antithrombin-III (AT-III) and thrombin

c. Catalyzes activity of heparin co-factor II, a secondary inhibitor of thrombin.

LMWH

a. Inhibits Xa more than thrombin

	Standard Heparin	LMWH
Anticoagulation response to fixed doses	highly variable	more consistent
$\frac{1}{2}$ life	short	longer
Binding to plasma proteins, cells	much	little

DIAGNOSIS AND MANAGEMENT OF ACUTE DVT

Noninvasive testing using impedance **plethysmography** or **compression ultrasonography** (using high resolution real-time ultrasound equipment) have mostly replaced venography in the diagnosis of DVT. Compression ultrasonography is the most commonly used non-invasive diagnostic test, with or without duplex ultrasound that adds gated Doppler and color-coded Doppler technology, which facilitates finding the veins to be studied.

Compression ultrasonography

1. Accurate in diagnosis of symptomatic DVT
2. Only 50% of symptomatic calf vein DVT's detected
3. Insensitive to asymptomatic calf vein DVT

Table 11.4
Diagnostic Approach Approach to Suspected DVT

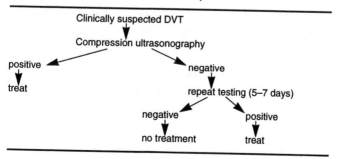

4. By monitoring symptomatic calf vein DVT's over 7 to 10 days, clinically important extension (to popliteal vein or above) can be detected

Current approach to the management of DVT is based upon the following observations (Table 11.4):

1. DVT in veins distal to the popliteal vein seldom embolize.
2. Fifteen to 25% of symptomatic calf vein DVTs will extend into the popliteal vein or beyond in 7 to 10 days. There is a significant risk of pulmonary embolism when this occurs.
3. By monitoring symptomatic calf vein DVTs for 7 to 10 days, extension can be detected and thus treated if it occurs.

Diagnosis of Recurrent DVT

The diagnosis of a recurrent DVT is often difficult because:

1. Two-thirds of episodes of symptoms suggestive of recurrence of DVT are not due to a new clot.
2. Non-invasive testing is less sensitive and specific after a previous DVT. It is helpful to have follow up after an acute DVT with non-invasive testing, at 3 to 6 months, to establish baseline results for comparison in case recurrent symptoms develop.

The following are **guidelines** for the diagnosis and treatment of a recurrent DVT:

1. A postacute DVT test is available, reveals no clot, and current testing is positive.
2. If the current test reveals extension of clot in previously positive veins.
3. If the current test is positive but unchanged, the decision to treat or not has to be based on less-than-reliable clinical features (degree of swelling and pain, risk factors, etc.).

TREATMENT
Standard Heparin
Route of Delivery

Continuous IV therapy and intermittent sub q therapy are probably equal in terms of efficacy. Bleeding complications are slightly more common with the sub q route. Both methods need monitoring of the degree of anticoagulation, however, the sub q route is difficult to monitor. Intravenous heparin results in an immediate effect, whereas there is a delay of around 3 hours before anticoagulant effect is achieved after initiating sub q treatment unless an initial IV bolus is given.

Achieving an appropriate level of anticoagulation within 24 hours of the onset of therapy is important. Various regimens for heparinization are used. Although it is appealing to use a regimen that takes into account the patient's weight, it has not been proven to be more beneficial than a standard dose with alterations made after close monitoring.

It is clear that the historical practice of administering a 5000 u bolus, followed by 1000 u/hour is inadequate for rapidly achieving a therapeutic range in many patients.

Heparin Dose

Sub q
Initial 5000 u bolus IV along with
17,500 u sub q repeated every 12 hours
Monitor PTT at 6 hrs. Goal 1.5–2.5 times control

IV
Method I.*
80 u/kg push followed by 18 u/kg/hour
PTT 6 hrs later:

<1.2 × C	same bolus + 4 u/kg/hr
1.2–1.5 × C	½ bolus + 2 u/kg/hr
1.5–2.5 × C	OK
2.5–3 × C	2 u/kg/hr
>3 × C	hold 1 hr, then 3 u/kg/hr

The PTT should be checked at 6 hr after each dose change.

---

*Raschke RA, et al. Ann Intern Med, 1993;119:874.

Method II.[*]

5000 u IV bolus followed by 1300 u/hour

PTT 6 hrs later:

$<1.2 \times C$	5000 u bolus, 1500 u/hour
$1.2-1.5 \times C$	2500 u bolus, 1400 u/hour
$1.5-2.5 \times C$	OK
$2.5-3 \times C$	to 1200 u/hour
$>3 \times C$	hold 1 hour, then to 1150 u/hour

The PTT should be checked at 6 hr after each dose change.

---

[*]Hirsh J, Weitz JI. Venous Thrombolism. In: Hoffman R, Benz EJ, Shattil SJ, Furie B, Cohen HJ, Silberstein LE, eds. Hematology: Basic Principles and Practice, 2nd ed. New York: Churchill Livingstone, 1995:1840.

Length of Heparinization

Studies show equal efficacy with 4 to 5 day heparin treatment and 9 to 10 day treatment Patients with large pulmonary emboli (PEs) should probably be treated for at least 7 days.

Low Molecular Weight Heparin

Currently (Spring 1996) LMWF is not FDA-approved for the treatment of established venous thrombosis, but likely to be in the near future. Because it has a longer half life and a standard dose/effect relationship, it can be given sub q once or twice daily without monitoring. Also, there are data to suggest that heparin-associated thrombocytopenia is less frequent with LMWH.

COUMADIN
When to Start?

Start coumadin 10 mg/day 24 hours postinitiation of heparin. It is believed that coumadin can even be started at the same time as heparin.

Monitoring

If the PTT is $<2.5 \times$ C, the PT can be used to monitor the coumadin dose. If the PTT is elevated beyond that range the PT will be elevated by the heparinization.

When to Stop Heparin?

No matter what the PT, patients should be continued on heparin at least 4 days post starting coumadin.

Goal

For most situations in the treatment of venous thromboembolism, an INR of 2–3 is recommended. For patients with recurrent venous thromboembolism an INR of 3–4 is reasonable.

Coumadin for How Long?

Length of anticoagulation remains controversial, but is classically 3 to 6 months for uncomplicated thromboembolism. The following are suggested lengths of anticoagulation.

Clinical Setting	Length of Treatment
Reversible risks	Shorter (6 weeks)
Non-reversible risks	Longer (6 months or more)
Idiopathic thrombosis	Longer (6 months or more)
Postop thrombosis	Shorter (4 weeks)

THROMBOLYTIC THERAPY

The indications for thrombolysis in patients with acute venous thrombosis remain controversial. Most agree that PE with hemodynamic compromise is an indication and many feel that young people with large proximal DVTs and no contraindication to therapy are good candidates for treatment, as well as patients with upper extremity DVT. Whether more patients with proximal DVT will have a better long-term clinical outcome with initial fibrinolytic treatment requires further study.

Suggested Reading

Dalen JE, Hirsh J, eds. Third ACCP Consensus Conference on Antithrombotic Therapy. Chest 1995;108:225S–231S, 305S–371S.

Hirsh J, Weitz JI. Venous Thrombolism. In: Hoffman R, Benz EJ, Shattil SJ, Furie B, Cohen HJ, Silberstein LE, eds. Hematology: Basic Principles and Practice, 2nd ed. New York: Churchill Livingstone, 1995: 1829–1842.

Schulman S, Rhedin AS, Lindmarker P, et al. A comparison of six weeks with six months of oral anticoagulant therapy after a first episode of venous thromboembolism. N Engl J Med 1995;332:661–665.

Chapter 12

Blood Transfusion

TREATMENT OF ANEMIA

Remember the following when considering the need for red cell transfusion:

1. When anemia develops gradually, a number of compensating processes occur which diminish symptoms: shift of O_2 dissociation curve, various cardiovascular adjustments, and an increase in plasma and total blood volumes. The elderly patient with a treatable, slowly developing chronic anemia (e.g., pernicious anema, iron deficiency), asymptomatic at rest, is best treated without transfusion. Volume overload (pulmonary edema) from transfusion is common in this situation.

2. Indications for transfusion in the above setting include:
   a. Angina pectoris
   b. Ischemic EKG changes
   c. High output congestive heart failure
   d. Organic cerebral symptoms
   e. Inability to keep the patient sedentary

3. Rapid bleeding may result in significant loss of blood volume without a drop in hematocrit. Beware of the patient with gastrointestinal bleeding and a normal hematocrit. Transfuse early.

Red Cell Components

Whole Blood

This component is used infrequently. It is primarily indicated for the actively bleeding patient who needs urgent volume replacement in addition to red blood cells (RBCs). Less acute bleeding (e.g., blood loss from surgery or mild gastrointestinal bleeding) can be managed by transfusion of packed cells.

Red Blood Cells (RBCs)

Prepared from freshly drawn blood allowing preparation of plasma components (e.g., cryoprecipitate) and platelet units. Packed cells stored in CPDA-1 have a shelf life of 35 days and a hematocrit of 70–80%. Packed cells stored with additive solutions (AS) have a shelf life of 42 days and a hematocrit of 50–60%. Remember there is appreciable plasma (albumin) left in this component. Packed cells given rapidly to the patient with a chronic anemia can precipitate **pulmonary edema.**

Leukocyte-Reduced RBCs

These preparations are indicated primarily to avoid chills and fever from **leukoagglutinin reactions** in multiply transfused patients or multiparous women. Leukocyte-reduced RBCs are indicated for future transfusions in patients who have experienced two febrile transfusion reactions (many patients experiencing one febrile reaction will not experience another). In addition, they may help to prevent **alloimmunization** in patients destined to receive multiple transfusions of blood products in the future (ongoing large trial to determine effectiveness). Leukocyte-reduced RBCs are also effective in reducing transmission of **cytomegalovirus.**

   The most efficient method of removing leukocytes is with the use of special filters. Filtration (1) may occur in the blood bank shortly after collection before processing of components, (2) may be done in the blood bank just before delivery for transfusion, or (3) may be done at the bedside at the time of transfusion.

Washed RBCs

Washed RBCs are indicated in patients experiencing allergic reactions secondary to plasma proteins (e.g. patients with congenital absence of IgA who have been sensitized to IgA). This component may also be used to remove complement from blood transfused to patients with cold agglutinin hemolysis.

Frozen Red Cells

Frozen blood allows for a long storage life. It is useful for storing rare blood types and collecting blood for autotransfusion in the rare blood type-patient scheduled for elective surgery. It is no longer used as a source of leukocyte-reduced RBCs.

PLATELET COMPONENTS

As discussed in Chapter 8, the treatment of thrombocytopenia differs with the mechanism. Platelet transfusions are generally reserved for severe production thrombocytopenia and are mainly used in the support of patients undergoing intensive chemotherapy. Available components include:

Random-donor Platelets

Prepared from a single unit of fresh blood by centrifugation techniques and concentrated in 50 ml of donor plasma. This product has a storage life of 3 to 5 days. In a 70 kg adult, 1 unit of random-donor platelets will raise the platelet count around 6,000/ul measured 1 hour post-transfusion. Increments are decreased in the setting of splenomegaly, infection, fever, DIC, or alloimmunization. The usual recommendation when transfusion is indicated is to give one unit of random-donor platelets per 10 kg body weight. The blood bank will pool platelets (commonly 6 units pooled) prior to delivery to the transfusion location. Platelets should be transfused within 4 hours of pooling. If volume overload is a problem (6 units of pooled platelets would be in a volume of 300 ml), platelets can be volume-reduced by centrifugation (100 ml final volume) by the blood bank.

Preferably platelets should be ABO-compatible, but non-ABO-compatible platelets can, and frequently are, used (probably slightly less recovery). ABO compatible platelets should be substituted if platelet responses are poor. Platelet concentrates contain some red cells so that Rh (D) immunoglobulin should be given to Rh-negative patients (especially young women) receiving platelets containing Rh-positive red cells.

Single-donor Platelets

Platelets are harvested by apheresis techniques from a single donor. May be effective in patients who demonstrate they are refractory to random-donor platelets secondary to alloimmunization. Comparable to 6–8 units of random-donor platelets.

HLA-Matched Platelets

Single-donor platelets obtained by apheresis from a human leukocyte antigen (HLA)-matched donor, indicated in the multiply transfused patient who has become sensitized to platelet antigens (primarily HLA antigens), and who no longer achieves a significant rise in platelet count with transfusion of random platelets. Such platelets are sometimes given to prevent sensitization in the patient who will require future platelet transfusion support. Human leukocyte antigen-identical platelets are usually obtained from a sibling by apheresis. Platelet numbers comparable to 6–8 units of random-donor platelets may be harvested in 2 to 3 hours from a donor. Patients may be supported through severe aplasia by platelets harvested from a single donor, donating three times a week.

Appropriate Use of Platelet Transfusions

- Patients with clinical bleeding secondary to thrombocytopenia (platelet count less than 50,000/ul and usually less than 20,000/ul).
- Prophylactically in patients undergoing invasive procedures with platelet counts less than 50,000.
- Practice has changed to some degree in recommendations for the prophylactic use of platelet transfusions in patients not undergoing invasive procedures (usually oncology patients undergoing intensive chemotherapy). Previously, platelets were given for counts less than 20,000/ul. Now since many patients (especially stable patients without bleeding sites) do not bleed even at lower platelet counts, transfusion is medicated primarily for the patient who is bleeding.

- Bleeding secondary to platelet dysfunction in some settings (p. 103)

OTHER COMPONENTS
Fresh Frozen Plasma (FFP)

Plasma is separated from fresh blood within 8 hours and frozen. It has a shelf life of 1 year. Fresh frozen plasma maintains activity of labile coagulation Factors V and VIII. Routine **single-donor plasma** contains other coagulation factors (including prothrombin complex Factors II, VII, IX and X). It is stored at 4°C and is stable in storage for long periods. However, the blood bank usually only stores single-donor plasma as FFP. Note that heat-treated plasma products such as "plasma protein fraction" do not contain coagulation factors.

Large volumes of FFP are usually required to correct coagulation abnormalities; volume overload is a problem. It is difficult to correct the PT and PTT to less than 1.5 times control because of the volumes required. The usual dose is 15+ml/kg given as rapidly as possible without precipitating a volume overload, which is difficult in many clinical settings.

Indications:

1. Treatment of dilution coagulopathy in the massively transfused patient, but only if a coagulopathy develops. The prophylactic use of FFP in this setting is discouraged
2. Rapid correction of the coagulation abnormalities in the patient on warfarin
3. Treatment of various congenital coagulation factor deficiencies (e.g., Factors II, V, VII, X, XI, XIII deficiency)
4. TTP, liver disease with bleeding, acute DIC
5. Initial treatment of Protein C and Protein S deficiency

Cryoprecipitate

Plasma separated from fresh blood is rapidly frozen at −90°C and then allowed to warm slowly at 4°C. Once rewarmed, most of the plasma is removed. A gelatinous precipitate is left suspended in a few milliliters of plasma, and the unit is stored at −20°C or less (shelf life, 1 year). A unit of cryoprecipitate contains an average of 100 units of Factor VIII (VIII:C), von Willebrand Factor multimers (around 50% of the activity in the original unit of plasma), and 200–250 mg of fibrinogen. Factor XIII and fibronectin are also present. Appropriate indications for cryoprecipitate include:

1. Treatment of hemophilia A (Factor VIII deficiency). Used less frequently since the development of successful viral inactivation procedures for Factor VIII concentrates.
2. Treatment of von Willebrand's disease.
3. Treatment of hypofibrinogenemia or dysfibrinogenemia.
4. Treatment of Factor XIII deficiency.

SOME COMMON TRANSFUSION PROBLEMS ENCOUNTERED BY THE HOUSE OFFICER

An Urgent Need for Blood for a Patient Who Is Exsanguinating

When there is not enough time to complete a crossmatch, the blood bank will supply type-specific (ABO and Rh) blood. Remember that this requires a properly labeled cross-match tube. It will take less than 5 minutes to determine the ABO and Rh type of the patient. The physician will have to sign a release stating the blood is needed as an emergency before a crossmatch can be completed (the latter takes 45 minutes to 1 hour to complete).

Uncommon Blood Type, Urgent Need

The blood bank may not have enough AB-negative, AB-positive, B-negative blood, etc., to fulfill the needs of an exsanguinating trauma patient. Here one may have to use blood that is not the patient's type. The following is a guide:

1. AB-negative patient:

O-negative blood is preferable. AB-positive, A-positive, B-positive, or O-positive blood may be used if there is time to complete a cross-match to rule out the possibility of prior Rh sensitization from a necessary previous transfusion of Rh-positive blood. Remember that, once the Rh-positive blood has been transfused to an Rh-negative recipient, sensitization is likely (less so in severely ill cancer patients on chemotherapy), and future transfusion with Rh-positive blood must be avoided.

2. AB-positive patient: Any type may be used. O-positive and A-positive are likely to be the easiest to obtain.
3. B-negative patient: O-negative blood is preferable. B-positive and O-positive may be used with the cautions mentioned above.

Notification by the Blood Bank That the Patient Has a Positive Direct Coombs' Test

See Chapter 4.

Notification by the Blood Bank That the Patient Has a Positive Antibody Screen with Crossmatching Difficulties

See Chapter 4, p. 41.

COMMON TRANSFUSION REACTIONS
Hemolytic Reactions

Immediate hemolytic transfusion reactions are quite rare and are usually due to errors in patient or blood identification (or both). Classical features include:

- Reaction early during the transfusion.
- Arm pain, chest pain, chills and fever and shock are characteristic; however, there may only be chills and fever.
- Intravascular hemolysis with hemoglobinemia and hemoglobinuria (p. 37).
- Acute renal shutdown is common with severe hemolytic reactions.

Delayed Hemolytic Transfusion Reactions

Delayed hemolytic transfusion reactions are classically seen several days following transfusion. They are caused by an anamnestic immune response to a minor RBC antigen to which the patient has previously been sensitized. Hemolysis is usually extravascular and less dramatic than in acute reactions.

Febrile Reactions (Table 12.1)

Such reactions, due to the presence (usually in the recipient) of HLA antibodies and subsequent activation of cytokines, e.g., IL-1, IL-6, TNF, are common, especially in multiply transfused patients. Symptoms such as chills and fever occur classically late in transfusion. Such reactions are not usually dangerous and respond to anti-inflammatory agents. They are decreased by using leukocyte-reduced blood products in those patients with a prior history of such reactions.

Approach to Febrile Reactions

The physician's dilemma when faced with a "chills and fever" transfusion reaction involves the difficulty in ruling out the presence of a hemolytic reaction. The following procedure is recommended when encountering a patient experiencing chills and fever while receiving a transfusion:

1. Discontinue the transfusion.
2. Doublecheck the patient's and the blood unit's identification.
3. Obtain a urine and plasma specimen to check for color (red or brown) indicative of hemoglobin or methemoglobin.
4. Return the unit and post-transfusion crossmatch specimen (and urine sample) to the blood bank.

Table 12.1
Transfusion Reactions

	Hemolytic	Leukoagglutinin
Incidence	Rare (1 in 10,000 transfusions)	Common (3% of all transfusions)
Classic clinical features	Arm pain, chest pain, back pain, shock, diaphoresis; may be only chills and fever	Chills and fever
Time of symptoms	Early in transfusion	Late in transfusion
Plasma/urine	Red (brown); free hemoglobin	Normal
Fatality	10%	Almost never fatal

5. Begin treatment for a presumed hemolytic transfusion reaction if:
   a. The urine/plasma color suggests hemoglobin. Hemoccult testing of the urine may help, but remember that the test is very sensitive to the presence of any red cells. Serum and plasma samples are almost always contaminated with red cells.
   b. The patient manifests any of the other symptoms/ signs suggestive of a hemolytic transfusion reaction (Table 12.1).
   c. Blood bank re-crossmatching indicates an incompatibility.

Most chills and fever reactions are due to **leukoagglutinins.** It may not be unreasonable to continue the transfusion in the following situations:

1. An identification check reveals the correct unit is hanging, and the patient is known to have had previous febrile non-hemolytic reactions with transfusions, and
2. The reaction is mild and occurring toward the end of the transfusion, and
3. The patient's transfusion history is well known to his physician, and
4. The plasma and urine reveal no evidence of hemoglobin.

However, one must be extremely careful and should err on the side of caution when confronted with minor transfusion-associated symptoms.

It is important to recognize that most febrile reactions do not reoccur with additional transfusions. One should not order leukocyte reduced blood for subsequent transfusions until a febrile reaction has been seen in two separate transfusions unless the initial reaction is quite severe.

Treatment of a Suspected Hemolytic Reaction

1. Draw bloods for a CBC, a coagulation screen (DIC is common), baseline renal function tests, electrolytes, and for blood bank re-crossmatching purposes (the patient will probably need further transfusion).

2. Give mannitol (or another diuretic) in an attempt to maintain urine output to at least 100 ml/hour.
3. Be prepared to treat hypotension, renal failure, etc.

Volume Overload

Such reactions still remain the most common serious hazard of transfusion. Be careful in the elderly patient or the patient with a history of congestive heart failure, especially if the anemia has developed slowly.

THE DANGERS OF TRANSFUSION

Transfusions are dangerous. Hemolytic, leukoagglutinin and allergic reactions may occur. The recipient may become sensitized to a minor RBC antigen leading to future difficulty in finding compatible blood. Volume overload may occur (especially in the elderly patient with heart disease and chronic anemia). Infection remains a major concern. Although there are rare cases today of contaminated blood, or the transfusion of blood from donors with malaria, babesiosis, etc., the major concern continues to be the transfusion of virus-infected blood.

Transfuse only when absolutely necessary. Encourage patients scheduled for elective surgery to undergo phlebotomy for autologous transfusion.

Suggested Reading

Beutler E, Masouredis SP. Preservation and clinical use of erythrocytes and whole blood. In: Beutler E, Lichtman MA, Coller BS, Kipps TJ, eds. Williams Hematology. 5th ed. New York: McGraw-Hill, 1995:1622–1643.

Menitove JE, Gill JC, Montgomery RR. Preparation and clinical use of plasma and plasma fractions. In: Beruler E, Lichtman MA, Coller BS, Kipps TJ, eds. Williams Hematology. 5th ed. New York: McGraw-Hill, 1995:1649–1663.

Murphy S. Preservation and clinical use of platelets. In: Beutler E, Lichtman MA, Coller BS, Kipps TJ eds. Williams Hematology. 5th ed. New York: McGraw-Hill, 1995:1643–1649.

Welch HG, Meehan DR, Goodnough ST. Prudent strategies for elective red blood cell transfusion. Ann Intern Med 1992;116:393.

Chapter 13

Polycythemia

One should consider the possible presence of polycythemia (increased total red blood cell volume) in a man with a persistent hematocrit greater than 55% and in a woman with a persistent hematocrit greater than 50%. Remember decreased plasma volume may result in an elevated hematocrit as well.

It is important to make a diagnosis of polycythemia primarily because of the therapeutic implications of a diagnosis of **primary polycythemia (polycythemia vera).** Table 13.1 contrasts primary and secondary polycythemia.

APPROACH TO WORKUP OF AN ELEVATED HCT

The following is offered as a logical stepwise approach to the evaluation of an elevated HCT:

1. Are any clinical features suggestive of **polycythemia vera** (P vera) present?
   - **Itching** (especially after a hot shower)
   - History of arterial **thrombosis**
   - **Splenomegaly**
   - **Elevated WBC**
   - **Basophilia**
   - **Elevated platelet count**
   - Abnormal **platelet morphology** on smear
2. If any of the above are present, particularly splenomegaly, thrombocytosis, or leukocytosis, a diagnosis of polycythemia vera is suggested and the physician should complete the workup:

Table 13.1
Comparison of Primary and Secondary Polycythemia

	Polycythemia Vera	Secondary Polycythemia
RBC mass	↑	↑
WBCs	Usually ↑	Normal
Basophils	Usually ↑	Normal
Platelets	Usually ↑	Normal
Platelet morphology	Usually abnormal	Normal
Spleen size	Usually ↑	Normal
Leukocyte alkaline phosphatase	Usually ↑	Normal
Serum B_{12}	Usually ↑	Normal
Itching	Common	Not seen

- **RBC mass**
- **Leukocyte alkaline phosphatase (LAP)**
- **Vitamin B_{12} level**

A bone marrow examination is not absolutely necessary but may be helpful. It classically reveals hypercellularity of all marrow elements and the absence of iron on a marrow iron stain.

3. If none of the above features is present, polycythemia vera is unlikely. The most likely etiologies are:

   a. **Decreased plasma volume.** Acute dehydration without an increase in RBC mass is a common explanation.

   b. **Hypoxia.** By far the most common etiology of secondary polycythemia. Pulmonary function studies and oxygen desaturation on blood gas determination may be diagnostic.

   c. **Stress polycythemia** (Gaisböck's syndrome, smoker's polycythemia). An elevated hematocrit is commonly seen in middle-aged males who smoke, are typically plethoric and hypertensive, and have none of the clinical features of polycythemia vera. The RBC mass is usually normal (high normal) and the plasma volume is decreased. Many do not consider this a syndrome, but rather one end of the normal bell-shaped curve. Remember that smoking alone will elevate the hematocrit because of the formation of carboxyhemoglobin.

4. If none of the above explanations fit, and if the hematocrit is persistently elevated, the physician should document the

presence of polycythemia with an RBC mass determination. If elevated, investigation for one of the less-common causes of polycythemia should be undertaken:

a. **Erythropoietin-producing tumors.** Renal cysts are most common with hypernephroma and hepatomas the next most-common etiologies.

b. **Methemoglobin, sulfhemoglobin** (nitrates in well water, congenital methemoglobinemia, rare).

c. **Hemoglobinopathy** (e.g., hgb. Chesapeake). The oxygen dissociation curve is shifted to the left with resulting tissue ischemia and secondary increase in erythropoietin (rare).

d. **Cyanotic heart disease.**

e. **Carboxyhemoglobin.** As mentioned above, smoking can raise the hematocrit several percentage points.

f. Mild erythrocytosis occurs in 10% of patients **post-renal transplant** [usually transient, sometimes responsive to angiotensin converting enzyme (ACE) inhibitors or theophylline].

TREATMENT
Secondary Polycythemia

For the most part no specific treatment is directed toward the polycythemia. Phlebotomy is rarely indicated in severe pulmonary hypoxemia or congenital heart disease. Treatment should be directed at the underlying etiology: stopping smoking; improving pulmonary function; eliminating nitrate exposure; treatment of the underlying tumor or cysts, etc.

Polycythemia Vera
Phlebotomy

The mainstay of treatment is phlebotomy to a normal RBC mass. It is important to phlebotomize to iron deficiency (low MCV) to eliminate an ongoing need for frequent phlebotomy. The objective is to keep the hematocrit less than 45% and the MCV in the iron-deficient range. It is useful to check the RBC mass periodically to make sure it is normal, as thrombotic complications of this disease correlate better with the RBC mass than the HCT.

Marrow Suppressive Agents

The Polycythemia Vera Study Group results indicate that $_{32}$p and chlorambucil treatment in P vera (given with the objective of normalizing the platelet count) decrease the incidence of thrombotic events but both (especially chlorambucil) increase the incidence of leukemia, lymphoma, and non-hematologic malignancies. Thus there is a therapeutic dilemma in P vera. Younger patients should probably be treated with phlebotomy alone. Older patients who have a higher incidence of thrombosis, especially during the first few years after diagnosis, fare better when treated with phlebotomy plus a marrow suppressive agent. **Hydroxyurea** is the most commonly used agent to control the platelet count in the older patient with P. vera or the younger patient who has clinical complications with an HCT controlled by phlebotomy. Interferon and anagrelide are also treatment options.

Other Treatment

Patients with severe **pruritus** may be helped by H_1 blockers and H_2 blockers, but pruritus may be refractory to all treatment approaches. Patients with **hyperuricemia** are at risk for gout and should be treated with allopurinol. ASA is relatively contraindicated because of the platelet dysfunction in P. vera. However many patients can tolerate ASA without bleeding.

Surgery

It is clear that surgery in the uncontrolled polycythemia vera patient is quite hazardous (bleeding and thrombotic complications). The RBC mass should be normalized before any major surgical procedure, preferably for 2 to 3 months prior to surgery.

Suggested Reading

Berk PD, Goldberg JD, Donovan PB. Therapeutic recommendations in polycythemia vera based on Polycythemia Study Group protocols. Seminars in Hematology 1986;23:132–143.

Hoffman R, Boswell HS. Polycythemia vera. In: Hoffman R, Benz EJ, Shattil SJ, Furie B, Cohen HJ, Silberstein LE, eds. Hematology: Basic Principles and Practice. New York: Churchill Livingstone, 1995:1121–1142.

Wasserman LR, Gilbert HS: Surgery in polycythemia vera. N Engl J Med 1963;269:1226.

Chapter 14

White Cells: Quantitative Abnormalities

When confronted with an abnormal WBC, the physician should first calculate the absolute count of each of the peripheral blood white cell forms to determine precisely the abnormality that needs to be explained.

Calculation of Absolute Counts (Table 14.1)

Absolute count = total WBC x differential % of individual cell types. This should be determined for:

- Granulocytes
- Neutrophils
- Eosinophils
- Basophils
- Lymphocytes
- Monocytes

The accuracy of absolute counts determined by this method is poor when cells represent fewer than 5–10% of all the white cells (e.g., eosinophils, basophils), and special direct counting techniques are needed if accuracy is important (e.g., eosinophil counts in asthma).

NEUTROPHILIA (TABLE 14.2)
Definition

Absolute neutrophil count greater than 8,000 per ml.

**Table 14.1
Normal Absolute Counts (Adults)**

Neutrophils	1,800–8,000/µl
Eosinophils	0–600/µl
Basophils	0–200/µl
Lymphocytes	1,000–5,000/µl
Monocytes	0–800/µl

Mechanism

Most neutrophilias are due to increased marrow proliferation. However, **redistribution** of cells among the various body neutrophil pools is the explanation for some neutrophilias. For example:

- **Acute stress** (exercise, endogenous or exogenous steroids, epinephrine, sepsis) causes a shift of cells out of the marrow into the peripheral blood and a redistribution of cells from the marginal pool (cells sequestered in the microcirculation and along blood vessel walls which are not counted by the WBC) to the counted peripheral circulating pool.
- **Chronic steroid administration** causes a decreased exodus of peripheral neutrophils to the tissues and neutrophilia.

Neutrophilic Leukemoid Reactions

"Leukemoid" refers to a persistent high WBC (usually neutrophilia) suggestive of leukemia. Counts may reach 50,000–100,000 cells per µl, and occasionally counts greater than 100,000

**Table 14.2
Common Causes of Neutrophilia**

Most causes of acute and chronic inflammation
Stress (emotional and physical)
Infections
Tumors
Drugs (steroids, epinephrine, lithium)
Splenectomy
Hemorrhage
Hemolytic anemia
Convulsions
Myeloproliferative disorders

Table 14.3
Comparison of CGL and Leukemoid Reaction

	Leukemoid Reaction	CGL
Total count	Usually < 100,000/μl	May be > 300,000/μl
Degree of left shift	Minimal	Large (blasts may be seen)
Basophils	Normal	Increased
Splenomegaly	Usually absent	Usually present
Leukocyte alkaline phosphate staining	Increased	Decreased or absent

per μl are seen. Infection, inflammation, and tumors are the usual causes. The type of leukemia usually suggested by a neutrophilic leukemoid reaction is chronic granulocytic leukemia (CGL) (Table 14.3).

Neutrophil Morphology in Infection

The individual neutrophil morphology on a peripheral smear in patients with a bacterial infection may be characteristic (must be a finger stick preparation as anticoagulant may spuriously cause similar changes):

1. **Toxic granulations** (coarse cytoplasmic granules). This is a nonspecific finding and may be seen in inflammation, cancer, and other conditions as well.
2. **Döhle bodies** (sky blue cytoplasmic inclusions). Sometimes the whole cytoplasm takes on a muddy, light blue color. More specific than toxic granulations but not pathognomonic of infection.
3. **Cytoplasmic vacuoles** (single or multiple and may be seen in only a small percentage of the cells). Reasonably specific for a bacterial infection. Anticoagulant will cause vacuoles, so the preparation must be a finger stick. Note that monocytes may have vacuoles normally, even on.

EOSINOPHILIA (TABLE 14.4)
Definition

Absolute eosinophil count greater than 600 μl. Note that direct counting methods are more accurate when the eosinophil percentage is less than 5–10%.

Table 14.4
Common Causes of Eosinophilia

Parasites
Allergic reactions (including drugs)
Dermatitis
Hodgkin's disease
Myeloproliferative disease
Adrenal insufficiency
Chronic renal disease
Radiotherapy
Drugs
Collagen vascular disease

In general, diagnostic evaluation of mild eosinophilia is not fruitful, but total eosinophil counts greater than 2,000 per μl can usually be explained. Massive eosinophilia may be seen in a very rare group of disorders known as the **hypereosinophilic syndromes.**

BASOPHILIA (TABLE 14.5)
Definition

Basophils are found easily on the peripheral smear and represent more than 1–2% of the differential. The presence of increased numbers of basophils may be particularly helpful as a diagnostic clue to the presence of a myeloproliferative disorder.

Table 14.5
Common Causes of Basophilia

Hypersensitivity reactions
Myeloproliferative disorders
  Polycythemia vera
  Agnogenic myeloid metaplasia
  Primary thrombocythemia
  CGL
Postsplenectomy
Inflammatory states

MONOCYTOSIS (TABLE 14.6)
Definition

Monocytosis is an absolute monocyte count greater than 800 per µl in an adult. The differential diagnosis of monocytosis is so extensive that its presence is generally not helpful in approaching the differential diagnosis of a clinical problem.

LYMPHOCYTOSIS (TABLE 14.7)
Definition

Lymphocytosis is an absolute lymphocyte count greater than 5,000 per µl. The experienced observer can usually distinguish between the morphology of the pleomorphic atypical lymphocytes seen in benign viral or allergic conditions and the abnormal lymphocytes seen in malignant lymphoproliferative diseases. In benign conditions the bone marrow usually does not show a significant lymphocytosis.

INFECTIOUS MONONUCLEOSIS SYNDROME

Infectious mononucleosis is an acute febrile illness seen primarily in teenagers and young adults; it is classically associated with **pharyngitis, lymphadenopathy, splenomegaly** and significant **atypical lymphocytosis.** Characteristic signs and symptoms are listed in Table 14.8. Remember the following:

Table 14.6
Common Causes of Monocytosis

Almost any inflammatory condition
Malignancy
SBE
Tuberculosis
Other infections
Collagen vascular disease
Myeloproliferative syndromes
Hodgkin's disease
Leukemias
Myelodysplastic syndromes
Neutropenia
During recovery from agranulocytosis

Table 14.7
Lymphocytosis, Common Causes

Normal morphology
  Pertussis
  Acute infectious lymphocytosis
  Chronic lymphocytic leukemia
  Waldenström's macroglobulinemia (sometimes normal morphology)
  Thyrotoxicosis
  Large granular lymphocyte disease
Atypical lymphocytes (nonmalignant)
  Infectious mononucleosis
  Cytomegalovirus infection
  Viral hepatitis
  Other viral illnesses
  Toxoplasmosis
  Typhoid fever
  Allergic reactions (drugs, etc.)
Abnormal morphology (malignant)
  Lymphosarcoma cell leukemia
  Acute lymphatic leukemia
  Mycosis fungoides, Sézary syndrome
  Hairy cell leukemia

1. The pharyngitis may be severe and is frequently accompanied by an exudate that is foul-smelling, rarely with some degree of respiratory obstruction.
2. Posterior cervical adenopathy is characteristic, but there may be generalized lymph node enlargement.
3. Ten to 15% of patients have an illness characterized by nonspecific malaise, fever, etc., without pharyngitis.
4. In the very young and the elderly, signs and symptoms are less specific, and pharyngitis is less common.
5. The course may be protracted, with nonspecific symptoms, lymphadenopathy, splenomegaly, persisting for weeks. Most patients are significantly improved by 3 weeks.

Basic Laboratory Features

White count: Usually elevated (between 10,000 and 20,000 per μl), with maximal counts occurring during the second and third weeks of the clinical illness.

Neutrophil count: Early in the course of the illness an ab-

Table 14.8
Signs and Symptoms of Infectious Mononucleosis

Common Symptoms	Common Signs	Percentage
Malaise	Adenopathy	(100%)
Warmth, chilliness	Pharyngitis	(85%)
Sore throat	Fever	(90%)
Myalgia	Splenomegaly	(60%)
Headache	Bradycardia	(40%)
Cough	Periorbital edema	(25%)
Anorexia	Palatal enanthem	(25%)

	Less Common Signs and Symptoms	
	Jaundice	(10%)
	Arthralgia	(5%)
	Skin rash	(5%)
	Diarrhea	(5%)
	Photophobia	(5%)

solute neutropenia is common, and occasionally neutrophil counts less than 500/μl are seen.

Lymphocytes: There is almost always an absolute lymphocytosis (greater than 5,000/μl) which is maximal during the second week of the clinical illness. At least 20% of lymphocytes have atypical morphology characterized by pleomorphism. The abnormal lymphocytes seen on smear are reactive T cells responding to infected host cells.

Hematocrit: Usually normal. Mild hemolysis may occur occasionally, and, rarely, severe Coombs' positive hemolysis is seen.

Platelet count: A mild thrombocytopenia, with counts greater than 100,000 per μl, is not unusual. A more severe thrombocytopenia, which may be immunologically mediated, occurs but it is quite rare.

Liver function tests: Mild liver enzyme abnormalities are common, and up to 50% of patients will show mild hyperbilirubinemia. Enzyme levels never reach the levels seen in viral hepatitis.

Cold agglutinins: Frequently elevated (without hemolysis) because of an antibody directed against the "i" red cell antigen.

Serologic Tests

Heterophil Antibodies

Heterophil antibodies are elevated in 90% of patients when the etiology is **Epstein-Barr Virus (EBV),** although elevation may not be detected until the third week of clinical illness. Differential absorption studies are necessary to identify the presence of those heterophil antibodies specific for infectious mononucleosis (absorbed by beef red cells but not guinea pig kidney cells).

Horse Cell Agglutinins (e.g., the "Monospot" test)

The use of horse red cells affords increased specificity over the use of sheep red cells. This is an excellent screening test for EBV infectious mononucleosis. Again, maximal positivity of the test occurs during the third week of the clinical illness.

Antibodies to EBV

The EBV is the etiologic agent in the infectious mononucleosis syndrome in the majority of cases. A number of serologic assays for specific antibodies to various antigenic components of EBV are available. They are primarily helpful in distinguishing EBV-positive, heterophile-negative infectious mononucleosis from the infectious mononucleosis syndrome due to other etiologic agents (e.g., CMV). They may also be useful in clarifying the etiology in patients with a recurrent infectious mononucleosis syndrome.

- IgM antibody to viral capsid antigen (**IgM anti-VCA**). Rises early in primary infection with EBV.
- IgG antibody to viral capsid antigen (**IgG anti-VCA**). Rises slightly later than IgM anti-VCA and remains detectable for life.
- Antibodies to the early antigen (**EA**) complex of EBV. Anti-EA antibodies arise later during the acute illness and may persist for life.
- Antibodies to Epstein-Barr nuclear antigen (**EBNA**). Anti-EBNA rise very late (months) after primary infection and are detectable for life.

One usually obtains IgG anti-VCA antibodies and anti-EBNA antibodies to diagnose EBV infectious mononucleosis. Anti-VCA is positive whereas anti-EBNA is negative.

Differential Diagnosis

Although a number of infections and even malignant conditions may mimic EBV+ and infectious mononucleosis, the following conditions are those most likely to give confusion:

1. **Cytomegalovirus infection.** Pharyngitis is much less common, as is lymphadenopathy. Fever and splenomegaly are common. It probably accounts for the majority of cases of EBV-negative mononucleosis. Unlike EBV (most Americans infected before age 25), only around 30% of Americans have been infected with CMV by age 20.
2. **Toxoplasmosis.** Pharyngitis does not occur and fever is uncommon. Most patients with acute infection present with lymphadenopathy (particularly posterior auricular). Diagnosis is usually established by the demonstration of a high IgM toxoplasmosis titer.
3. **Miscellaneous.** Included are bacterial pharyngitis, acute leukemia, infectious hepatitis, and other viral illnesses, including acute infection with HIV-I. Atypical lymphocytosis can be prominent in Hepatitis A and B.

Complications

Severe complications are quite rare:

1. **Neurologic.** Includes encephalitis, meningitis, peripheral neuropathy and the Guillain-Barre syndrome. Death has been reported, especially with the latter syndrome.
2. Occasional **superinfection** with bacterial infections has been reported, sometimes in association with agranulocytosis.
3. **Splenic rupture.** Death from spontaneous splenic rupture has been reported. Diagnosis is easy to miss. Be wary of a history of sudden, brief, sharp abdominal pain.
4. **Other,** rarely fatal, severe complications include myocarditis, hepatic necrosis, and airway obstruction.

Infection in the Immunocompromised Host

CMV infections in the **immunocompromised host** is a serious illness which can cause multiorgan damage (e.g., pneumonia in bone marrow transplant recipients; retinitis in AIDS; and gastrointestinal disease, retardation, and deafness in newborns). **Toxoplasmosis** can cause serious CNS infection in AIDS. **EBV** is an etiologic agent for Burkitt's lymphoma in African children and nasopharyngeal carcinoma in far east Asia. It can lead to malignant lymphoproliferative disease in the immunocompromised host. EBV has essentially been ruled out as the culprit for chronic fatigue syndrome.

NEUTROPENIA
Definition

An absolute neutrophil count in an adult, less than 1800 per μl. It should be noted that 1500 per μl is the lower range of normal in some studies and that 2% of a normal population will have counts less than these lower-limit values. Blacks may have a lower normal neutrophil count than Caucasians. "Granulocytopenia" is a synonym for neutropenia.

Neutrophils, Normal Lower Limits (varies with the lab)

Age	Count
1 month–10 years	1500/μl
>10 years	1800/μl
African Americans	1500/μl
>70 years	1800/μl (but less neutrophil response to infection and more neutropenia early in infection)

Risk of infection varies with the degree of neutropenia and the setting. Neutrophil counts greater than 1000/μl carry little extra risk; counts greater than 500/μl but less than 1000/μl are associated with some increased risk; counts less than 500/μl and especially less than 200/μl are dangerous, especially if persistent. Risk of infection is increased in severely neutropenic patients if monocytes and eosinophils are also decreased.

Defining the Mechanism

Persistent neutropenia, even of a mild degree, not obviously explained by an acute event (such as a viral infection), must be evaluated and a specific etiology defined if possible.

Routine Database

- CBC
- Bone marrow aspiration and biopsy
- Evaluation of spleen size (PE, sonogram or CT scan)
- Review of peripheral smear (finger stick)

The above data should help to place the neutropenia into one of the following categories as to **mechanism:**

- Decreased bone marrow proliferation
- Ineffective bone marrow production
- Decreased neutrophil survival
- Redistribution neutropenia (margination)

Decreased Bone Marrow Proliferation

Common Etiologies

- Aplastic anemia
- Marrow infiltration (myelophthisis)
- Drug-induced neutropenia or aplasia

The bone marrow reveals a decrease in granulocyte precursors and may indicate a specific etiology in the case of marrow-infiltrative diseases such as leukemia, metastatic cancer, etc. A drug-induced etiology is most common.

Drug-induced Hypoproliferative Neutropenia

a. **Universal, Dose-Related**

Most of the chemotherapeutic agents used in oncology cause a dose-related neutropenia (and usually thrombocytopenia) in everyone. Other agents, not usually thought of as marrow-suppressive, will cause neutropenia in everyone if used in large enough doses. These include:

- Chloramphenicol
- Ethanol
- Rifampin

b. **Idiosyncratic, Dose-Related**

These drugs cause neutropenia only in some individuals. Usually the drug has to be taken in large doses for a period of time (at least 2 weeks) prior to the onset of neutropenia. Unrecognized host factors are a prerequisite. The best studied drug in this category is **chlorpromazine,** which is known to inhibit DNA synthesis. Neutropenia usually develops during the first 3 months of therapy or not at all. The neutropenia is usually mild (may be severe), and the white count rapidly reverts to normal after discontinuation of the drug. **Other** less well-studied **agents** that may fall into this category of drug-induced neutropenia include:

- Antithyroid agents
- Other phenothiazines
- Imipramine hydrochloride
- Antibiotics
- Chloramphenicol
- Sulfonamides
- Carbenicillin
- Isoniazid
- β-lactam antibiotics
- Phenylbutazone
- Penicillamine

c. **Hypersensitivity Reactions**

Some drug-induced neutropenias appear to be allergic, hypersensitivity reactions, suggesting an antibody mechanism (usually not adequately proven). Such reactions do not appear to be dose-related and are frequently accompanied by eosinophilia. Neutropenia may occur anytime, but classically occurs early in the course of treatment with a drug to which there has been previous exposure. The reaction appears to be more common in women, the elderly, and in patients with allergic histories. Drugs reputed to give this type of reaction include:

- Sulfonamides
- β-lactam antibiotics (eosinophilia, rash and fever-common)
- Gold

- Chloramphenicol
- Penicillins
- Phenylbutazone
- Quinidine
- Procainamide
- Diuretics (thiazides, ethacrynic acid)
- H_2 blockers
- Antithyroid drugs
- Captopril
- Methyldopa
- Hydralazine
- Allopurinol
- Clozapine
- Ticlopidine
- Phenytoin
- Carbamazepine
- Tolbutamide

Acute *Agranulocytosis.*
Severe, isolated, drug-induced production neutropenia with an absolute neutrophil count less than 200 is known as **acute agranulocytosis.** It is seen primarily with idiosyncratic drug reactions and is life-threatening. Recovery usually occurs within 2 weeks of discontinuing the drug. Treatment involves recognition, discontinuation of all possible offending drugs, and hospitalization and broad-spectrum antibiotic coverage for fever or other signs of infection. The usefulness of **granulocyte colony-stimulating factors** is anecdotal, but they are frequently used in severe cases.

Aplastic Anemia. Acute agranulocytosis is a short, self-limited illness with complete recovery if the patient survives the short neutropenia period. In contrast, aplastic anemia, which may occur as a hypersensitivity reaction to certain drugs, is usually chronic and often fatal. Bone marrow transplantation has become the procedure of choice for the young patient with severe aplasia and the availability of a HLA-identical sibling. Androgens may occasionally be useful in the patient with mild aplasia.

In vitro bone marrow culture techniques are available and

may be useful to distinguish cases caused by nonimmune stem cell damage from those caused by immunologic stem cell suppression. This latter mechanism is found in patients with autoimmune disease and is frequently T lymphocyte-mediated. Responses may be seen with steroids, antithymocyte globulin, plasmapheresis, splenectomy, etc.

Ineffective Bone Marrow Production
Common Etiologies

- **Megaloblastic anemia**
- Folate deficiency
- B_{12} deficiency
- Drugs which interfere with folate metabolism (methotrexate, hydroxyurea, cytosine arabinoside, pyrimethamine, diphenylhydantoin)
- **Myelodysplastic syndromes**

The bone marrow is cellular but discloses qualitative abnormalities usually of all cell lines. There is intramarrow cell death and frequently peripheral cytopenia. In B_{12} and folic acid deficiency the peripheral neutropenia rapidly corrects with appropriate vitamin treatment.

Decreased Neutrophil Survival.

Some patients with autoimmune disease such as SLE and Felty's syndrome have chronic neutropenia secondary to antineutrophil antibodies. Some drug-induced neutropenias may also be secondary to autoantibodies to peripheral neutrophils. In vitro detection of **antineutrophil antibodies** is difficult; the multiple available tests suffering from problems of specificity. The bone marrow in such patients is cellular, but usually reveals only early precursors ("maturation arrest" picture), the more mature cells being released to the peripheral circulation early.

Such a mechanism for leukopenia, even when severe, is usually less dangerous and life-threatening than production neutropenias of the same degree. **Remember:**

- The peripheral pool of granulocytes is quite small in comparison to the marrow pools.

- Cells pass through the peripheral pool rapidly (in a few hours) on their way to the tissues.
- A neutrophil count, therefore, gives little information pertinent to the important issue—the number of cells being delivered to the tissues.
- Be more concerned about severe neutropenia with a hypoplastic bone marrow (agranulocytosis, aplastic anemia).
- Be less concerned about severe neutropenia with a hypercellular bone marrow.

Redistribution Neutropenia

Normally the peripheral blood granulocytes are distributed about equally between a **"circulating pool"** of cells measured by the peripheral neutrophil count and a **"marginal pool"** of cells distributed along vessel walls, in the microcirculation, and in the spleen (not counted by the neutrophil count). Cells may shift from the circulating pool to the marginal pool, giving a false impression of neutropenia in the following circumstances:

- Hypersplenism
- Overwhelming bacterial sepsis
- Viremia

Tissue delivery of neutrophiles is frequently adequate even though the peripheral neutrophil count suggests otherwise. Bone marrow granulocyte precursors are adequate or increased.

LYMPHOPENIA
Definition

An absolute lymphocyte count of less than 1000 per μl is usually considered abnormal, although in one series 6% of a normal population had counts less than 1000 per μl. Lymphocytopenia has little diagnostic significance and is often unexplained. Known associated conditions include:

- Congenital immunologic deficiency syndromes
- Malignancy
- Hodgkin's disease

- Chemotherapy
- Radiotherapy
- Collagen vascular disease (lupus)
- Inflammation
- Corticosteroid excess
- Uremia
- Acute alcoholism
- AIDS

Suggested Reading

Dale DC. Neutropenia. In: Beutler E, Lichtman MA, Coller BS, Kipps TJ, eds. Williams Hematology, 5th ed. New York: McGraw-Hill, 1995: 810–815, 824–828.

Lichtman MA. Classification and clinical manifestations of neutrophil disorders. In: Beutler E, Lichtman MA, Coller BS, Kipps TJ, eds. Williams Hematology, 5th ed. New York: McGraw-Hill, 1995:810–815.

Loughran TP, Starkebaum G. Large granular lymphocyte leukemia. Medicine 1987; 66:397.

Waterbury L, Zieve PD. Selected illnesses affecting lymphocytes. In: Barker LR, Burton JR, Zieve PD, eds. The Principles of Ambulatory Medicine, 4th ed. Baltimore: Williams & Wilkins, 1995:624–628.

Zacharski LR, Linman JW. Lymphocytopenia: its causes and significance. Mayo Clin Proc 1971; 46:168.

Index

Note: Pages followed by f indicate illustrations; those followed by t refer to tables.